Eating For Health™
Your Guide to Vitality & Optimal Health

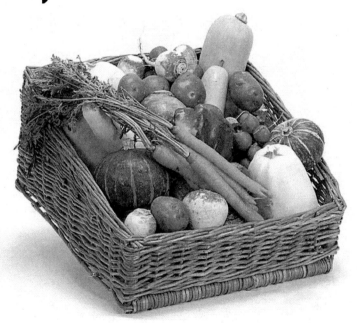

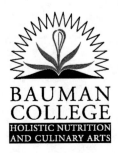

BAUMAN
COLLEGE
HOLISTIC NUTRITION
AND CULINARY ARTS

©2008   *Eating For Health™ Your Guide to Vitality and Optimal Health*

Editorial: Edward Bauman, M.Ed. Ph.D. and Mindy Toomay
Cover Design and Cover Photos: Chris Clay Bauman
Book Design: Magnolia Studio

ISBN: 978-0-6151-9456-1

BAUMAN COLLEGE
P.O. Box 940
Penngrove, CA 94951

EMAIL: info@baumancollege.org
WEB: www.baumancollege.org
PHONE: 800-987-7530
FAX: 707-795-3375

Table of Contents

Table of Contents

The Two Pots

Chinese Folk Tale as told by
Olga Voronina, Vitality Fasting™
staff and massage therapist

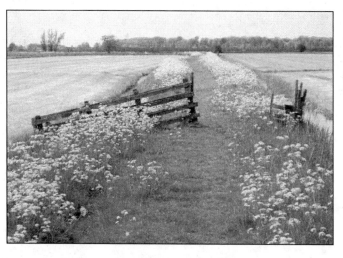

An elderly Chinese woman had two large pots, each hung on the ends of a pole, which she carried across her neck.

One of the pots had a crack in it while the other pot was perfect and always delivered a full portion of water, at the end of the long walk from the stream to the house. The cracked pot arrived only half full.

For a full two years this went on daily, with the woman bringing home only one and a half pots of water. Of course, the perfect pot was proud of its accomplishments. But the poor cracked pot was ashamed of its own imperfection, and miserable that it could only do half of what it had been made to do.

After two years of what it perceived to be bitter failure, it spoke to the woman one day by the stream. "I am ashamed of myself, because this crack in my side causes water to leak out all the way back to your house."

The old woman smiled, "Did you notice that there are flowers on your side of the path, but not on the other pot's side? That's because I have always known about your flaw, so I planted flower seeds on your side of the path, and every day while we walk back, you water them. For two years I have been able to pick these beautiful flowers to decorate the table. Without you being just the way you are, there would not be this beauty to grace the house."

Each of us has our own unique flaw. But it's the cracks and flaws we each have that make our lives together so very interesting and rewarding. You've just got to take each person for what they are and look for the good in them.

SO, to all of my friends, have a great day and remember to smell the flowers on your side of the path!

Ed

PART ONE:
Eating For Health™

Walk into any good book store and take a look at the nutrition section. You will find an absurd number of diet books — all putting forth different theories, all competing ferociously for your dollars. How many of these authors have a genuine concern for the long-term health of their readers?

Sadly, the focus of most of these books is on weight loss solely for the sake of looking like a movie star. Can the science of nutrition really be so limited and so two-dimensional?

Eating For Health™ is a way of life. It reflects a relationship to food based on consciousness, gratitude, sound science, and positive energy. Unlike the stultifying glut of extreme and unbalanced diet approaches currently pumped into the marketplace, the *Eating For Health*™ model is a beacon in the fog to those weary of yet another potential diet failure.

As a nutrition strategy, the *Eating For Health*™ model is adaptable to building, balancing, or cleansing goals. This is a unique feature that allows individuals to customize a plan that accounts for "The Four Cs": Constitution, Context, Condition, and Commitment.

This model is the foundation of your nutrition practice, on which your clients' diets are rebuilt. It is a powerful tool based on both cutting-edge research and plain common sense.

Eating For Health™:
A New System, Not Another Diet
by Edward Bauman, M.Ed., Ph.D.

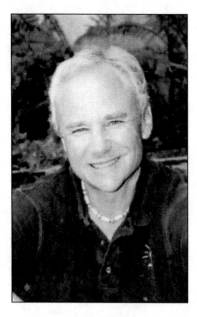

Many people come to me and ask, "What diet is right for me? Is it the Zone, Atkins, Ornish, Pyramid, or Blood Typing? I need to lose weight, gain energy, and get fit. I've tried and failed so many diets that I am ready to give up, but I can't. I feel lousy and look worse. I've turned my mirrors inside out to no avail. I am raging about my aging. I need help!"

For the past 25 years, I have been guiding people of all ages and stages of life with a myriad of health problems: some cosmetic, many life threatening. To address the wide range of issues my clients face, I devised a system — not a diet — called *Eating For Health*™ (E4H).

Each one of us has unique genetic tendencies, needs, tastes, and tolerances, all of which should be factored into a customized food and nutrition plan. One size does not fit all when it comes to proper nourishment.

We all need differing amounts of healthful foods and nutrients to cope with a fast paced, stress-filled, and toxic world. Similarly, our metabolism is challenged to continually adapt to changes in seasons, situations, climate, and health challenges. It stands to reason that what we ate as children, a mediocre *Standard American Diet* (SAD), will not nourish us as aging adults.

Change is the one constant in our lives. Let's investigate how to change for the better and improve our health by supporting our metabolism, brain function, and ability to self-heal. Cleaning up the diet by clearing out the debris in our pantries, refrigerators, and medicine cabinets is a good start. Finding out how to shop for, prepare, and enjoy healthy foods is the key that unlocks the door to your rejuvenation.

A map can help you find your destination in the most direct way. Therefore, a great step forward on the path to nutritional wellness is to meet with a professional Nutrition Consultant to receive an in-depth assessment and analysis of your individual situation. If you are struggling with one or more health issues, the consultant can review and evaluate the latest research and advise you on the specific therapeutic foods, herbs, and nutrients that will support your healing.

You are the co-creator in the E4H process. Consider the foods that were nourishing and healing for you in the past, as well as the foods you currently rely on for energy or emotional gratification Some of these foods are probably loaded with caffeine, bad fats, and sugar — ingredients that will sabotage you when the momentary distraction wears off, pleasure fades, and disease takes over.

Proper nutrition is a major form of health investing. It is safer than the stock market as a hedge against the risk of illness. When you eat poor quality food, you are dipping into the nutrient reserves in your bones, soft tissue, organs, glands, skin, and hair. You wear the results of being overdrawn nutritionally — an unhealthy appearance, and feel the warning signs of ill health — fatigue, pain, and mood swings.

Eating For Health™: A New System, Not Another Diet—CONTINUED

Vow to wake up and *Eat For Health* by choosing fresh, seasonal, chemical-free, nutrient-rich, organic foods that can replenish the reserves that have been drained by the poor quality foods you have been living on.

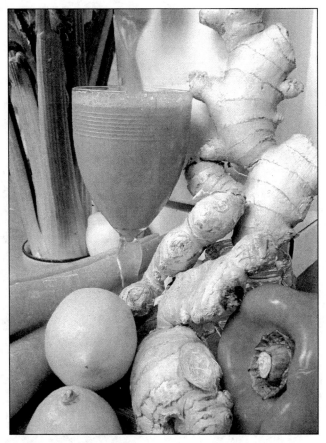

The usual suspects, also known as health banditos, are the stimulants, sugars, pastries, pastas, processed cheeses, artificial sweeteners, and margarine found in white-flour-laden, over-processed, frozen, microwaved meals served in restaurants or grabbed on the run. Such foods are formulated in laboratories to over-stimulate our taste receptors so that we are no longer satisfied by the crunch of a carrot, the refreshingly sweet juice of a fresh mango, or the zing of fresh garlic. While it's easy to overeat nutrient-poor, sugary, salty, greasy snack foods, you can enjoy naturally satisfying, nutrient-rich vegetables, grains, seeds, legumes, and lean proteins in abundance.

E4H is a whole foods approach to nutrition developed to provide an alternative to the USDA Food Pyramid and other unbalanced diet approaches, ranging from the protein-heavy Atkins Diet to Fruitarianism. The E4H model guides us in choosing nutrient-dense and diverse foods that are organic, local, seasonal, and unprocessed.

The goal of this unique system is to provide optimal amounts of macronutrients (proteins, fats, and carbohydrates), micronutrients (vitamins and minerals), phytonutrients (plant alkaloids with protective value), and other vital factors (enzymes, tastes, energetic properties) that can be most efficiently digested and assimilated.

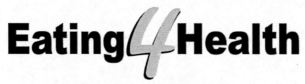

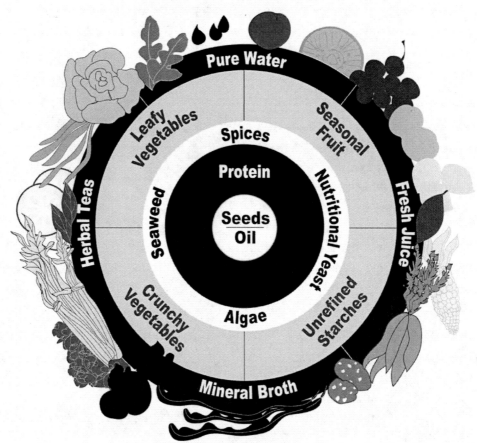

A Rejuvenating Food System
© by Edward Bauman, Ph.D.

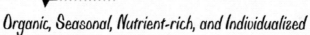

Organic, Seasonal, Nutrient-rich, and Individualized

	SEEDS/OILS	PROTEIN	LEAFY VEGETABLES	CRUNCHY VEGETABLES	UNREFINED STARCHES	SEASONAL FRUIT	BOOSTER FOODS
Daily Servings	2-3	2-4	1-3	1-3	2-4	2-4	2-4
Serving Size	1 Tbsp. oil 2 Tbsp. seeds	3 oz. animal 6 oz. vegetable	1 cup	1/2 cup	1/2 cup root vegetable, grains, bread.	1/2 cup or 1 med. piece	1 tsp. to 1 Tbsp.
Examples	Flax, sunflower, sesame, and almonds.	Poultry, fish, eggs, milk, and beans.	Salad mix, kale, and spinach.	Broccoli, string beans, cukes, onions, celery.	Yams, winter squash, corn, millet, rice.	Berries, apple, grape, and citrus.	Nuts, yeast, seaweed, algae, spices.

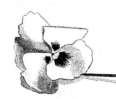
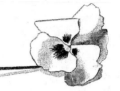

Eating For Health™ Guidelines
by Edward Bauman, M.Ed., Ph.D.

1. Increase intake of local, seasonal, fresh, organic foods.

2. Drink plenty of purified water each day, about 1/2 cup (4 ounces) every hour. To determine the total amount you need, divide your weight in half and drink that many ounces of water.

3. Read labels and avoid foods with artificial ingredients.

4. Decrease intake of refined and artificial sugars, white flour products, unnatural fats, added hormones, preservatives, colors, and antibiotics.

5. Diversify sources of proteins, fats, and carbohydrates.

6. Ingest 1 gram of protein per kilogram (2.2 lbs) of normal body weight.

7. Eat protein by ten in the morning and 1-3 more times during the day.

8. Eat protein to curb sugar cravings.

9. Minimize caffeine intake to 50mg or less (1 cup black tea, 3 cups green tea, or 1/2 cup coffee or espresso).

10. Eat more monounsaturated fat (olives, avocados, almonds) than saturated fat (animal, dairy, coconuts) or polyunsaturated oils (soy, corn, sunflower).

11. Decrease consumption of glutinous grains (wheat, rye, oats, barley) to prevent digestive disturbance and inflammation.

12. Increase consumption of gluten-free grains (rice, corn, millet, quinoa, buckwheat, amaranth), which are mineral rich and easy to digest.

13. Increase consumption of leafy (e.g. kale), crunchy (e.g. broccoli) and starchy (e.g. yam) vegetables to provide abundant minerals.

14. Eat three portions of vegetables in a meal to 1 serving of protein and 1 serving of fat for pH balance.

15. If body temperature is cold, eat more proteins, essential fatty acids, seaweeds, and warming spices such as ginger and cayenne.

16. If body temperature is warm, eat more cooling foods, such as fruits, vegetables, and green herbal teas and spices like mint, rosemary, lemongrass, and rooibus.

17. Determine a diet direction according to your metabolic tendency: Building if metabolism is fast, Cleansing if metabolism is slow, or Balanced if metabolism is neither fast nor slow.

18. Add booster foods to the diet to increase energy, detoxification, and antioxidant activity.

19. Undertake a simplified diet or fasting program seasonally, including colon cleansing and increased spiritual practice.

20. Enjoy your food and let others eat in peace.

Thanks for working on your health and sharing this important information.
Blessings and Peace to All!

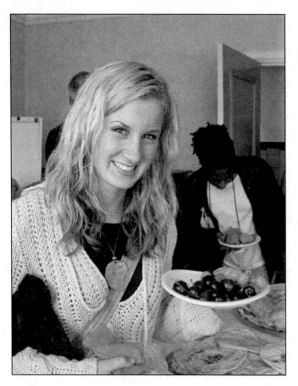

The Four Levels of Eating

by Edward Bauman, M.Ed., Ph.D.

Eating For Health™ is a process, rather than a method. To differentiate E4H from other food systems, I developed the concept of the *Four Levels of Eating*. Each level has its place and reflects the awareness and maturity of a person when he or she iseating, a behavior that affords us abundant choice and delight but is often done with little thought. To create sustainability in one's own and the planet's health, we need to exercise greater levels of thought, awareness, and discrimination around food selection.

Now let's visit the *Four Levels of Eating*.

Level One: Eating for Pleasure

This level is an immature and impulsive approach to eating, aimed at maximizing pleasure and minimizing pain. Eating at this level is for immediate gratification. "I ate it because it tasted good" and "I ate as much of it as wanted to" are hallmarks of this stage.

Refined sugar and flour, dairy products, and unhealthy fats are in this category. Food choices typically reflect what we were fed as young children to quiet and appease us, such as ice cream, cookies and milk, candy, and soft drinks. Excessive coffee, alcohol, or chocolate is also Level One eating. Emotional eating, which often means compulsive overeating, is a Level adaptation to pain, tension, and stress.

Level Two: Eating for Energy

Blood sugar regulation drives one's food choices at this level. We choose substantial foods that allay hunger. The goal is to fill up and not have to eat again for three to four hours.

In Level Two, carbohydrates become more complex; breads may have some whole wheat in them, but are still refined. Fast foods like burgers and burritos are common choices. Little concern is placed on the quality of the food, the likely nutrient loss due to processing, possible pesticide residues, environmental toxins, or added hormones, antibiotics, coloring, and artificial flavors. Animal proteins, peanut butter, breads, pastas, chips, and pizza are common Level Two foods. Fresh fruits and vegetables play a minimal role in the diet at this stage.

This is a highly acid-forming, allergy-inducing, and clogging diet pattern. Level Two eaters are typically unconcerned with the ecological impact of their food choices.

The Four Levels of Eating—CONTINUED

Level Three: Eating for Recovery

The inevitable cumulative effects of Level One and Level Two eating are poor body composition — frequently obesity — and diminished energy, health, and brightness of mood.

People experiencing these effects often go on a diet formulated by someone else that organizes foods into good and bad categories and limits quantities. It may or may not emphasize high-quality, organic foods. Examples of Level Three eating are diet plans such as the Zone, Atkins, Ornish, Weight Watchers, Food Combining, Blood Typing, and Raw Foods.

The benefits of such diets are typically short-lived. There is an immediate positive effect from eating fewer refined and processed foods, but then we reach a point of diminishing return. The diet is no longer satisfying and no longer producing the promised effects. The tendency then is to stay with the rigid, reductionist approach even longer or to slip back to Level One or Level Two eating patterns.

This is a more mature approach than the first two levels, but it can be tiresome, judgmental, and sometimes supplement driven.

Level Four: Eating for Health

The goal of this approach is lifelong learning about optimum nutrition, the healing effects of foods, and an aesthetic and spiritual approach to the culinary arts. It shares some qualities with Level Three, but allows for more personal choice, variety, seasonality, and individuality according to one's personal needs, tastes, ethnic origin, and commitment level.

Food choices at Level Four are not made by formula, but rather by discerning what the body needs and what the best available choices are at a given time. At this level, we choose among a wide variety of healthy, organic foods. We exercise moderation in the amount of foods we eat, and take more time and care in its preparation and presentation. Food is understood and appreciated as an instrument of personal healing and sharing with community. Nourishing ourselves becomes a wise, mature, and loving act of awareness cultivated through daily practice.

The *Eating For Health*™ model provides a map for healthy eating that draws on many different systems and philosophies, including Traditional Chinese Medicine, Ayurveda, naturopathy, cutting-edge biochemistry, and ecological sustainability.

It was designed to help nutrition professionals guide their clients toward the most nutritionally sound approach for them as individuals. By eating well consistently, they learn what foods best nourish and sustain them during stressful changes that threaten health and impede recovery.

In *Eating For Heath*™, we embrace two powerful maxims – "food is the best medicine" and "know thyself" — and create a synergy that opens the way to wellness and service.

The Joy of Conscious Eating

by Edward Bauman, M.Ed., Ph.D.

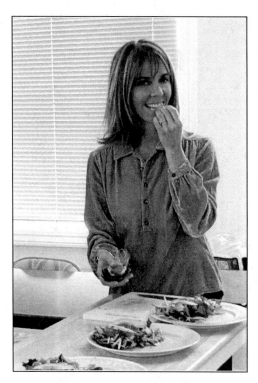

My intention is to create a culture of health based on a conscious diet, balanced lifestyle, and consideration for the earth. The process of changing from non-nutritive, disease-promoting foods to highly nutritive, health-promoting foods begins with making a firm commitment to change and generating support from family and friends. The next step is finding a good place to buy healthy foods, like natural health food stores or local farmers markets. Step three is learning to prepare *Eating For Health™* meals.

Finally, and the toughest step to master, is choosing healthy treats instead of dips, sodas, pastries, or sugary confections. Snacks, and even desserts, can be both nutritious and delicious if we choose a piece of fresh, organic, seasonal fruit with a handful of sunflower or pumpkin seeds, or a homemade oatmeal date cookie.

Often when we eat for pleasure rather than for health, it is because our inner children are calling out for love. We equate foods made of sugar, flour, milk, and/or chocolate with love, which obviously they are not.

Old habits direct us to reach for a quick fix — a café latte, perhaps — to alleviate our failing blood sugar. The symptoms of low blood sugar include fatigue and mental dullness. These states can be avoided if we eat well-timed, nutrient-rich meals based on: a wide variety of fresh vegetables; high-quality proteins such as cold water fish, free-range poultry, or eggs; and whole grains, legumes, and seeds. Purified water and herb tea are the healthiest beverages to drink, replacing sugar-saturated sodas and bottled fruit juices. Attitude is also important. Slow down and enjoy your meals. Give thanks and reflect.

You will notice that when you are more deliberate in choosing what and how to eat, a new level of stability and consistency will emerge in your energy level and moods. Two important tips are to start the day with foods that nourish you and to plan one good meal ahead.

The following keys to success with "conscious vs. convenience" eating are simple habits to practice daily until they become second nature:

- ▶ Slow down while eating;
- ▶ Chew your food thoroughly;
- ▶ Don't allow yourself to become distracted while you are eating;
- ▶ Eat below the level of fullness;
- ▶ Give thanks for your food and your life; and
- ▶ Continue to expand the variety of seasonal foods in your diet.

From Fast Foods to Fad Diets... To Eating For Health™

by Edward Bauman, M.Ed., Ph.D.

The health of a majority of Americans is worsening as you read this. Why? To state the obvious, we all have too much stress in our lives and not enough time to exercise, eat right, and relax.

One result of the typical, out-of-balance modern lifestyle is that our childhood desires for foods that are soft, sweet, and creamy or salty, crunchy, and greasy have become the preferred standards of cuisine for many adults. I call this epidemic "fork and mouth disease," sold to us in our youth by television and marketing and established in our brains as a reliable pleasure provider. It is no surprise that we are witnessing an unprecedented rise in obesity, blood sugar imbalances, and irrationality in our culture and the world.

Fast Foods are False Foods

The loss of health, firm body composition, and vitality experienced by huge numbers of children and adults alike is due to the huge quantities of processed, refined, adulterated, and synthetic foods we Americans so proudly consume. Fast foods — as documented thoroughly in *Fast Food Nation* by Eric Schlosser and *Crazy Makers* by Carol Simontacchi (see bibliography) — are made from the least expensive ingredients possible and are loaded with chemicals, damaged fats, artificial ingredients, and flavor enhancers. Fast foods are stimulating without being nourishing, but they are certainly profitable.

Their low prices appeal to millions of people with a lack of funds and little regard for health. Junk food marketers target children as young as three years old and in 2002 spent an estimated $15 billion in children's marketing alone.

> *"Americans now spend more money on fast food than on higher education, personal computers, computer software or new cars."*
>
> Eric Schlosser, *Fast Food Nation*

Current research correlates fructose intake not only with obesity, but also with cardiovascular disease, due to its elevating effect on our blood fats, particularly triglycerides. Yet in 1970, high fructose corn syrup replaced refined sugar as the sweetener of choice for manufacturers, due to its low cost and claims to be non-insulin stimulating, and therefore a "healthy" sugar.

Don't be fooled by the word "fructose" on food labels. The fructose in an apple is a far different substance than the white powder that is poured into soft drinks, pastry products, and thousands of packaged foods and beverages. The apple is rich in vitamins, minerals, and fiber, whereas fructose powder is totally devoid of the nutrients needed for proper blood sugar regulation. Fructose is processed in the liver as a chemical that increases oxidation, inflammation, and allergic response. These effects make it stimulating and debilitating at the very same time.

From Fast Foods to Fad Diets… To Eating For Health™—CONTINUED

High-protein Diets

Artificial or refined sugars combined with poor-quality or cooked fats is a recipe for weight gain, as well as brain chemistry alterations such as depression, insomnia, and anxiety. Sadly, people suffering from fatigue, weight gain, and mood disorders are susceptible to fad diets, medication, extreme exercise, and other unhealthy behaviors. Recreational drug use, alcohol abuse, and other aberrant behaviors are often used as coping devices by people who feel poorly.

The *Atkins Diet* has preyed on the overweight, moody, and exhausted by providing an alternative eating plan that tends to work for a short time. The diet calls for mostly protein and fatty foods, with little or no carbohydrates for the first two weeks. The carbohydrate exclusion forces the body to burn fat by a process called ketosis, which allays hunger and expedites weight and fat loss. After this "induction" period, dieters are allowed only minimal carbohydrates. The good news is that such high-protein diets all but eliminate refined and artificial sugars. So, what is the problem with them?

The bad news is that high-protein diets are often lacking in natural, unprocessed plant foods that deliver healthy doses of vitamins, minerals, and fiber and serve a variety of essential functions in the body. High-protein diet gurus often recommend numerous dietary supplements to make up for the deficits in their food plans. This is woefully inadequate, as most supplements are synthetic and therefore poorly absorbed, providing only limited and temporary benefits.

Another serious problem is that little attention is directed to the quality of protein and fat on the *Atkins Diet.* One can easily be a Taco Bell, McDonald's, and Baskin Robbins *Atkins Diet* eater. Mass-marketed animal foods tend to be loaded with bovine growth hormones, antibiotics, and pesticides that concentrate in the animal's fat tissues, writes John Robbins in *The Food Revolution.* These substances are not safe for daily consumption, yet they are frequently eaten by typical, non-organic Atkins dieters.

These folks may lose weight and experience a big boost of energy in the early stages of the diet, but they are also stressing their livers, kidney, and immune systems with antigens and carcinogens. With repeated ingestion, despite sometimes dramatic weight loss, these substances can expedite cancer or autoimmune disease. This is too great a life-long risk for the short-term benefits conferred. Relying on these unbalanced diet approaches to achieve weight loss typically leads to yet another diet failure.

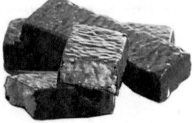

The *Atkins Diet,* and other programs that emulate it, are not long-term solutions to the chronic overeating of the wrong foods. It is true that foods such as refined flour products, breads, pastries, pasta, and desserts are eliminated while a person is on the *Atkins Diet.* However, a time eventually comes when most high-protein eaters plateau in their weight loss and become sluggish, moody, and as tired as before, only to "fall off the wagon" and return to refined carbohydrates. The short-term pleasure derived from eating donuts, a bag of cookies, or a heaping bowl of spaghetti is so great that many people cannot restrain themselves and revert back to their over-consuming ways.

From Fast Foods to Fad Diets... To Eating For Health™—CONTINUED

This suggests that an addiction to sugar and processed foods was always there and that the high-protein diet was a temporary fix, at best. Professional nutritional help is needed to provide education and support for carbohydrate addicts, which could be any of us reading this article.

The major flaw of the *Atkins Diet* is that many people, in their zeal to shed pounds, erroneously eliminate too many carbohydrates, thereby becoming deficient in much needed fluid, fiber, antioxidants, and trace elements found in complex carbohydrates. Another serious detriment of the high-protein, low-carbohydrate diet is its potential adverse effect on the acid/alkaline balance.

Protein foods, such as meat, fish, eggs, poultry, and dairy products are high in nitrogen and are therefore "acid forming." Over-consuming acid-forming foods creates *acidosis* (hyperacidity). The problem with this is that the blood, lymph, mouth, and small intestine need to maintain an alkaline predominance in order to carry out essential metabolic functions. Fruits, vegetables, herbs and non-glutinous grains — such as millet, quinoa and brown rice — are alkaline-forming and are the healthy carbohydrates generally missing from high-protein diets.

Susan Lark, MD, author of *The Chemistry of Success: Secrets of Peak Performance*, states that acid-forming diets contribute to a negative mineral balance that leads to degenerative conditions such as osteoporosis, arthritis, fibromyalgia, gout, liver and kidney disease. Continued high-protein intake will eventually strain the digestive system, create putrefaction in the gut, and overstimulate the immune system, which may begin to perceive excessive protein as *antigenic* (toxic) material. This is the birth of auto-immune disease.

A Healthier Approach

Natural foods are the basis for the *Eating For Health*™ approach. I created the *Eating For Health*™ model (see the chart on the page 4) to provide a bull's eye method for choosing a wide variety of whole, natural foods to satisfy numerous vital health needs. The overwhelming benefit is that a person can choose between many different healthy foods. Rather than reducing the amount and variety of foods consumed, *Eating For Health*™ encourages people to eat a plant-based diet, with no more than 50% of their protein coming from animal sources. This has ecological benefits to the soil, air, and water, as well as to one's digestive system. Careful attention to food quality, quantity, variety, and seasonality is the foundation of this approach.

Within an *Eating For Health*™ food plan, a person can build nutrient-dense meals including protein-rich foods and quality fatty acids. However, these are complemented by an equal or greater amount of whole grains and fresh vegetables, and are accented with condiments called booster foods, such as nutritional yeast, sea vegetables, algae, culinary herbs, and spices. Attention to colorful foods — such as red, orange, green, and yellow fruits and vegetables – is encouraged to provide ample antioxidants and alkaline minerals like calcium, magnesium, potassium, chromium, selenium, and zinc. The *Eating For Health*™

From Fast Foods to Fad Diets...To Eating For Health™—CONTINUED

eater chooses form a wide variety of satisfying foods, without overeating refined carbohydrates, protein, or suspect fats.

Switching from fast food to *Atkins* to *Eating For Health*™ is a journey of the soul, moving from the clutches of habitual patterns to the freedom of maturity, conscious choice, and regeneration. It takes time and, in most cases, the support of ateacher, classmates, and family is crucial.

It is a tragedy that people have to become sick before they wake up and take responsibility for what they put into their precious bodies. Hopefully, we are at the end of the era in which mass marketing and government subsidies support a climate of consumption that renders us vulnerable and without will or even hope, simply to put money in the pockets of the giants of agriculture, food production, and medicine. Eating fast food or being on unbalanced diets will not provide the nutritional support for our population to think clearly and change the way we live — personally, politically, economically, and ecologically.

Eating For Health™ holds great promise to reverse the illnesses that plague so many of our citizens. In time, as it becomes more widespread and people awaken to the perfect sustenance that nature can provide, a new era of health, prosperity, and spirituality can emerge, albeit amidst untold tons of fast food packaging and diet books decomposing in our landfills.

To eat whole, natural foods is a sign of recovery from an era of misinformation and gullibility. Spread the knowledge of what the body needs to grow and repair itself and do not be fooled by false claims of better living through chemistry. Nature is what sustains the planet and all its beings. Growing, buying, and consuming fresh, natural foods will bring optimal health to the body and healing to the earth.

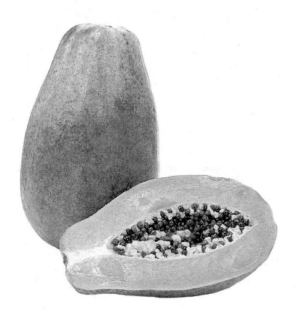

The Complete Eating For Health™ Program

SAMPLE DIETARY RECOMMENDATIONS

Seafood, vegetarian diet with therapeutic herbs and phytonutrients.

Breakfast

12 oz. fresh fruit juice made from:

- 6 green apples
- 1 lemon
- 1" piece fresh ginger root

With vitality boosters:

- 1 tsp. green powder (spirulina, chlorella, wheatgrass, and/or barley grass)
- 1 Tbsp. protein powder
- 1 Tbsp. ground flax seeds
- 1 oz. aloe concentrate
- 4 oz. fresh or frozen berries
- 4 oz. filtered water

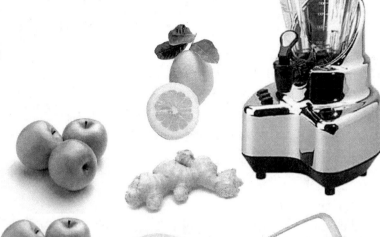

Lunch

1 cup cooked brown rice, millet, quinoa or buckwheat

1 1/2 cups dark green leafy salad greens

1/2 cup grated or chopped tri-colored seasonal vegetables

4 oz. soy tofu, 2 oz. soy tempeh

OR

4 oz. cooked lentils or garbanzo beans

OR

3 oz. steamed or baked salmon, tuna, halibut, sea bass, or swordfish

1 Tbsp. unpasteurized sauerkraut

1 Tbsp. hydrated sea vegetables (either hiziki, wakame, dulse, arame)

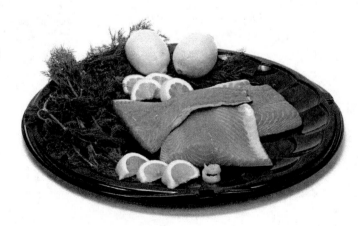

The Complete Eating For Health™ Program—CONTINUED

Afternoon Snack

12 oz. fresh organic vegetable juice made from:

    1 lb. carrots

    1 cucumber

    1 small beet

    1/2 cup fresh green herbs of choice

With vitality boosters:

    1 tsp. Vital Scoop (a blend of whey, flax, greens and fruit extracts)

    1 Tbsp. ground flax seeds

    1 oz. aloe concentrate

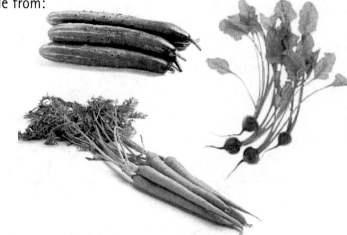

Dinner (by 6PM)

Baked yam, winter squash, or organic potato topped with:

    2 Tbsp. pumpkin seeds

    1 tsp. nutritional yeast

    4 oz. goat, soy, or organic cow yogurt

    OR

    2 oz. sheep feta cheese

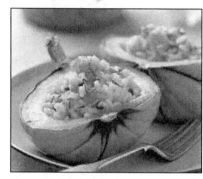

    1 cup steamed cruciferous vegetables (broccoli, cauliflower, cabbage, Brussels sprouts) cooked with

    1 large chopped onion

    4 cloves garlic

    1/2 tsp. turmeric or curry powder

Seasonings may include:

    Bragg's Liquid Amino's Sauce®

    Tamari

    OR

    Savory herbal seasonings

Dessert (2 hours after a main meal)

1 cup fresh seasonal, organic fruit with:

    3 Tbsp. chopped almonds, walnuts, pecans, or cashews

    1/2 tsp. grated lemon, orange, or tangerine peel

    1/2 tsp. cinnamon, nutmeg, cardamom, and/or ginger powder

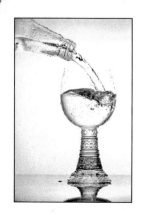

Beverages

Drink 3 liters of filtered water with lemon or designated herb tea blend.

Eating For Health™ Daily Diet Inventory

EATING FOR HEALTH	SERVINGS	FOOD CONSUMED		SERVINGS
SEEDS AND OILS:	2-3			
Flax: 2 Tbsp.				
Nuts: 2 Tbsp.				
Olive oil: 1 Tbsp.				
Avocado: 1/4				
PROTEINS:	2-4			
Poultry: 3 oz.				
Seafood: 3 oz.				
Eggs: 1				
Organic dairy: 1 glass milk				
Legumes: 6 oz. cooked				
Protein powder: 2 Tbsp.				
BOOSTERS:	1-4			
Yeast: 1 Tbsp.				
Algae: 1 tsp.				
Spices: 1 tsp.				
Seaweed: 1 Tbsp.				
FRUITS:	2-4			
1 piece or 1/2 cup				
VEGETABLES:	2-6			
Crunchy: 1/2 cup				
Leafy: 1 cup				
STARCHES:	2-4			
1/2 cup roots				
1 cup cereal				
2 slices bread				
BEVERAGES:	8 -12			
Water: 1 cup				
Herb tea: 1 cup				
Fresh juice: 1 cup				
Broth: 1 cup				
OTHER: Treats, snacks, etc.				

Eating For Health™ Investment Account

Name: _____ Date: _____

You have heard that you are what you eat. It's true! Likewise, what you eat is an investment in your health both now and in the future. Take an inventory of your dietary habits and choices to calculate your net nutritional worth. It will help you become more aware of how you can eat better, live longer and with much less distress. Consult with a nutrition professional for maximum benefit.

PART I: DAILY PROFIT AND LOSS CALCULATIONS

POSITIVE NUTRITION ASSETS 1 = <1/week 2 = 1–2/wk 3 = >2/wk	NEGATIVE NUTRITION LIABILITIES 1 = <1/week 2 = 1–2/wk 3 = >2/wk
1. ___ Organic (pesticide-free) food	1. ___ Conventionally grown food
2. ___ Fresh food	2. ___ Packaged food
3. ___ Whole foods	3. ___ Refined foods
4. ___ Local food	4. ___ Imported food
5. ___ Seasonal food	5. ___ Out of season food
6. ___ Homemade food	6. ___ Restaurant food
7. ___ Eating slowly	7. ___ Eat quickly
8. ___ Fruit and vegetable-based meals	8. ___ Meat, dairy or grain-based meals
9. ___ Essential fatty acids	9. ___ Saturated, transaturated fats
10. ___ Grass-fed free range meat and poultry	10. ___ Grain, hormone-fed meats
11. ___ Wild, cold water fish	11. ___ Farm fed fish
12. ___ Hormone, antibiotic free eggs (with Omega-3 fats)	12. ___ Commercial eggs
13. ___ Organic dairy products (milk, cheese, butter)	13. ___ Commercial dairy products
14. ___ Cultured dairy (yogurt, kefir, buttermilk)	14. ___ Uncultured dairy
15. ___ Organic soy products (non-GMO)	15. ___ Commercial GMO soy
16. ___ Organic legumes (lentils, peas, beans)	16. ___ Commercial legumes
17. ___ Organic whole grains (rice, millet, quinoa)	17. ___ Refined grains (bread and pasta)
18. ___ Natural sweeteners (honey, maple, Sucanat)	18. ___ White sugar, Nutrasweet
19. ___ Booster foods (nuts, yeast, algae, herbs, seaweed)	19. ___ Extra added sugar, salt, MSG
20. ___ Pure water, herb tea, fresh juices, broths	20. ___ Tap water, coffee, soda, black tea

_____ **Total Positive Nutrient Assets**	_____ **Total Negative Nutrient Assets**
_____ **Part I Net Nutrition Worth**	_____ **Circle Behavior Change Numbers**

Eating For Health™ Investment Account—CONTINUED

Now that you have completed Part I of the *Eating For Health™* Investment Account, you can reap additional health benefits from setting up your own IRA, which will further add to your nutritional reserves and provide important fuel for cellular cleansing and rejuvenation. The key is to increase your positive assets while decreasing your negative withdrawals. Enjoy the exercise and then put it into good use.

PART II: INDIVIDUAL REJUVENATION ACCOUNT (IRA)

POSITIVE IRA ACCOUNT 1 = <1/week 2 = 1-2/wk 3 = >2/wk	DEBIT WITHDRAWALS 1 = <1/week 2 = 1-2/wk 3 = >2/wk
1. ___ Hi-potency natural multiple. Supplement with herbs. (Comprehensive nutrition support.)	1. ___ Low potency synthetic. Multiple supplement. (Poor bioavailability.)
2. ___ Organic green food powder. (Nourishes the blood.)	2. ___ Commercial green food. (Pesticide-laden.)
3. ___ Organic whey, rice or soy protein powder. (Amino acid support.)	3. ___ Commercial vegan protein. (Incomplete protein.)
4. ___ Organic flax seeds. (Essential fatty acids and fiber.)	4. ___ Commercial flax more than 3 weeks old. (Oxidizes and rancid.)
5. ___ Buffered or Ester Vitamin C. (Detoxification and immune support.)	5. ___ Ascorbic Acid. (Made from corn syrup.)
6. ___ Natural Vitamin E (d-alpha or mixed). (Antioxidant, inhibits lipid peroxidation.)	6. ___ Synthetic Vitamin E (dl-alpha). (Oxidizes, rather than protects from free radical damage.)
7. ___ Natural calcium, magnesium. (Vitamin D, boron and HCl supplements Bone and nerve support.)	7. ___ Commercial calcium supplements. (Poor bioavailability.)
8. ___ Natural zinc/selenium/chromium, as needed. (Weight, immune, and blood sugar support.)	8. ___ One-A-Day vitamins. (Lacks trace minerals.)
9. ___ Targeted, appropriate herbal support. (Strengthens weak systems.)	9. ___ Tobacco, drugs, or more than 1 alcohol drink per day. (Increases toxic load.)
10. ___ Seasonal fasting. (Detoxification and rejuvenation.)	10. ___ Toxic exposures, poor diet, or overwork. (Acid forming.)

Part III: Positive IRA Assets _____ Debit ATM Withdrawals _____ Net IRA Value _____

Part I: Nutrition Worth _____ + Part II Nutrition Worth _____ = Total Nutrition Worth

Macronutrient Serving Size Chart

PROTEIN	SERVING SIZE*
DAIRY	
Cottage cheese (low fat)	1/2 cup
Yogurt (low fat)	1 cup
ANIMAL PROTEIN	
Eggs (whole)	2 large
Egg (whites only)	4 large
Meat (Lean)	2 oz.
Poultry	2 oz.
Wild game	2 oz.
Fish (cold water)	3 oz.
(salmon, mackerel, trout)	
Tuna, water packed	2 oz.
Sardines, in sardine oil	2 oz.
SOY AND LEGUMES	
Soy beans, tofu, lentils	6 oz.
Soy protein powder	1 oz.
Whey protein	1 scoop

Palm of hand or approx. 15g of protein.

FATS AND OILS	SERVING SIZE*
OMEGA-3 OILS	
Flax, pumpkin, walnut	2 tsp.
MONOUNSATURATED	
Olive	2 tsp.
OMEGA-3 SEEDS	
Flax, pumpkin, sesame, and sunflower	1Tbsp.
Avocado	1 Tbsp.
NUTS	
Walnuts, hazelnuts (w3)	1 Tbsp.
Almonds (w9)	1 Tbsp.
OTHER FATS	
Eggless mayonnaise	1 Tbsp.
Butter	2 tsp.

Approximately 6g of fats.

COMPLEX CARBOHYDRATES	SERVING SIZE*
PASTA	
Whole grain	1 cup
GRAINS	
Whole grains	1/2-3/4 cup
Whole grain bread	1 1/2 slices
VEGETABLES	
High starch veggies (15-20%)	1 cup cooked
High water, fiber veggies (3-6%)	1 1/2 cups
FRUITS	
Higher carb fruits (15-20%)	1/2 cup
Lower sugar fruits (3-6%)	1-1 1/2 cups

Approximately 20g carbohydrate.

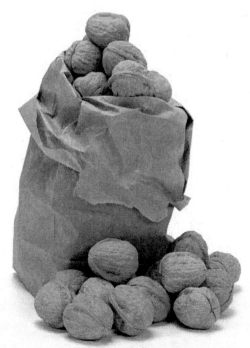

Eating For Health™ Shopping List

by Edward Bauman, M.Ed., Ph.D.

Hormone Free Meats!

Local, Seasonal, Organic When Possible!

EAT 3 servings of plants for each serving of animal!

Seeds, Nuts and Oils:

- ❏ Almonds
- ❏ Chia seeds
- ❏ Coconut oil
- ❏ Filberts
- ❏ Flax oil
- ❏ Flax seeds
- ❏ Hazelnuts
- ❏ Hemp oil
- ❏ Hemp seeds
- ❏ Nut butters
- ❏ Olive oil
- ❏ Pecans
- ❏ Pumpkin seeds
- ❏ Sesame oil
- ❏ Sesame seeds
- ❏ Sesame tahini
- ❏ Sunflower seeds
- ❏ Walnuts

Proteins:

Meats/Seafood:

- ❏ Chicken
- ❏ Fish
- ❏ Lamb
- ❏ Shellfish
- ❏ Turkey

Dairy:

- ❏ Free-range eggs
- ❏ Organic cheese
- ❏ Organic milk
- ❏ Organic yogurt

Legumes/Legume Products:

- ❏ Black beans
- ❏ Edamame *(fresh soy beans in pods)*
- ❏ Garbanzo beans
- ❏ Hummus
- ❏ Lentils (green and red)
- ❏ Pinto beans
- ❏ Tempeh
- ❏ Tofu
- ❏ White beans

Fresh Fruits

- ❏ Apples
- ❏ Apricots
- ❏ Bananas
- ❏ Berries
- ❏ Cantaloupes
- ❏ Figs
- ❏ Grapefruit
- ❏ Grapes
- ❏ Mango
- ❏ Nectarines
- ❏ Oranges
- ❏ Peaches
- ❏ Pears
- ❏ Pineapple
- ❏ Plums
- ❏ Pomegranate
- ❏ Rhubarb
- ❏ Watermelons

Booster Foods

- ❏ Arame seaweed
- ❏ Green algae
- ❏ Hijiki seaweed
- ❏ Nori seaweed
- ❏ Nutritional yeast

Herbs:

- ❏ Basil
- ❏ Dill
- ❏ Oregano
- ❏ Rosemary
- ❏ Sage
- ❏ Thyme

Sweet Spices:

- ❏ Allspice
- ❏ Cardamon
- ❏ Cinnamon
- ❏ Cloves
- ❏ Coriander
- ❏ Nutmeg

Savory Spices:

- ❏ Black pepper
- ❏ Cayenne pepper
- ❏ Chile pepper
- ❏ Garlic (granulated)
- ❏ Ginger
- ❏ Mustard powder
- ❏ Turmeric

Eating For Health™ Shopping List—CONTINUED

Fresh Vegetables

- ❏ Asparagus
- ❏ Avocado
- ❏ Beans
- ❏ Broccoli
- ❏ Brussels sprouts
- ❏ Burdock root
- ❏ Butternut squash
- ❏ Carrots
- ❏ Cauliflower
- ❏ Celery
- ❏ Corn
- ❏ Cucumbers
- ❏ Garbanzo beans (sprouted)
- ❏ Ginger
- ❏ Green onions
- ❏ Kale
- ❏ Lentils (sprouted)
- ❏ Lettuce
- ❏ Onions
- ❏ Peas
- ❏ Peas (sprouted)
- ❏ Peppers
- ❏ Potatoes
- ❏ Radishes
- ❏ Red cabbage
- ❏ Russet potatoes
- ❏ Shiitake mushrooms
- ❏ Squash
- ❏ Sweet potatoes
- ❏ Tomatoes
- ❏ Zucchini

Starches

Whole Grains

- ❏ Brown rice (short or long grain)
- ❏ Millet
- ❏ Oats
- ❏ Polenta
- ❏ Quinoa
- ❏ Whole grain cereal
- ❏ Whole grain sprouted bread
- ❏ Whole grain tortillas
- ❏ Wild rice

Root Vegetables and Winter Squash

- ❏ Beets
- ❏ Parsnips
- ❏ Pumpkin
- ❏ Squash
- ❏ Sweet potatoes
- ❏ Turnips
- ❏ Yams

Frozen Food Suggestions

- ❏ Berries
- ❏ Carrots
- ❏ Chicken breasts
- ❏ Corn
- ❏ Fish
- ❏ Green beans
- ❏ Mango
- ❏ Mixed vegetables
- ❏ Peas
- ❏ Tamales

Canned Food Suggestions

- ❏ Applesauce
- ❏ Artichokes
- ❏ Black beans
- ❏ Marinara sauce
- ❏ Pineapple
- ❏ Pinto beans
- ❏ Salmon
- ❏ Sardines
- ❏ Tomatoes (whole)
- ❏ Tuna

Beverages

- ❏ Almond milk
- ❏ Fresh fruit juice
- ❏ Fresh vegetable juice
- ❏ Green tea
- ❏ Herb teas
- ❏ Miso or chicken broth
- ❏ Rice milk
- ❏ Soy milk
- ❏ Water (pure)
- ❏ Water (sparkling)

Condiments

- ❏ Apple cider vinegar
- ❏ Agave
- ❏ Balsamic vinegar
- ❏ *Bragg's Liquid Aminos*
- ❏ Brown rice vinegar
- ❏ Fruit preserves
- ❏ Ginger (pickled)
- ❏ Honey
- ❏ Maple syrup
- ❏ Mustard
- ❏ Wasabi

Reassessing The Great Pyramid

by Edward Bauman, M.Ed., Ph.D.

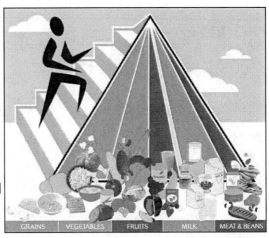

In the summer of 1992, the *U.S. Department of Agriculture* (USDA) gave us the Food Guide Pyramid as a graphical representation of federal dietary recommendations. This Pyramid had a broad foundation of carbohydrates at the bottom and a tiny capstone of fats at the top. We now have My Pyramid (www.mypyramid.gov) as the working model. While it is a good step forward, it still fails to address the qualitative issues of fresh, local, seasonal, and organic foods.

The USDA has "reassessed" the original pyramid — avoiding the word "revised" to quell perceptions that their food guide recommendations are far from health promoting. In the past decade, during which the Pyramid emphasized six to eleven servings per day of any carbohydrate, obesity has risen dramatically, causing nutritionists to question its wisdom. As Harvard nutritionist Walter Willett points out, "The pyramid treats all fats as bad, and all starches as good, which they clearly are not."

What's that sound? Those are the first notes sounding from the "Get a New Pyramid" bandwagon. Joining in is a host of critics who claim that the USDA, when creating the Pyramid, probably did some bending in order to please a powerful, deep-pockets lobby that wanted to keep the "Eat Lots of Bread" message prominently displayed. Enough of that criticism and the "Get a New Pyramid" bandwagon may eventually take on enough riders to make the cover of Time magazine.

Is conventional wisdom really wise? Sure it is. But conventions change, as does wisdom. Lately, I've noticed more reports of mainstream health care providers and nutritionists incorporating alternative medicine and diet concepts into their practices. I have yet to hear of an osteopathic physician who practices alternative medicine, however, crossing over to embrace mainstream pharmaceuticals. That is a bandwagon that will never get rolling.

Eating Irony

▶ The Japanese eat very little fat and suffer fewer heart attacks than the British or Americans.

▶ The French eat a lot of fat and also suffer fewer heart attacks than the British or Americans.

▶ The Japanese drink very little red wine and suffer fewer heart attacks than the British or Americans.

▶ The French and Italians drink large amounts of red wine and also suffer fewer heart attacks than the British or Americans.

CONCLUSION:

Eat and drink what you like. Speaking English is apparently what causes heart attacks.

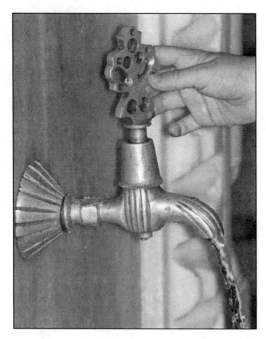

The Truth About Your Drinking Water

by Janice Hughes, Share Guide Editor

Nowadays, many people realize that tap water is not safe to drink. Californians, in fact, are the largest consumers of bottled water in the country. But if you talk to people and ask them about this issue, most can only give a vague explanation of the problem. They know that the water is not "safe," but they don't know exactly what toxins are in it, or where they come from.

The fact is that water contamination may be America's number one health problem. Over 70% of our body is water, and we need clean water every day to rejuvenate our system and flush out toxins. Water is the foundation of our health, and if the foundation is poor, the entire structure is jeopardized.

There are thousands upon thousands of chemicals used in our society, with approximately 1,000 new ones introduced each year. The Federal Safe Drinking Water Act regulates only 100 contaminants. How effective can that be? And congress is seeking right now to relax the regulations on water, not strengthen them.

A shocking statistic is that in 1992 and 1993 alone there were over 230,000 violations of the Federal Safe Drinking Water Act by public water systems. That's just for the few contaminants that are currently being regulated. The system has broken down, unable to cope with the by-products of our industrialized society.

The scary thing is that the bottled water many of us have turned to as a supposed "safe alternative" may not be clean either. While bottled water may taste better, there are no assurances that it is free of contaminants, because what most people don't realize is this: *bottled water is largely unregulated!* Many bottled waters with names that include words such as "mountain," "spring" and "crystal clear" are actually tap water that has been filtered through a very simple (and inadequate) filtration system to remove enough chlorine so that it tastes better. (Since you can't taste, see or smell most contaminants, they know you can't tell the difference.) And we won't even discuss the exorbitant prices we pay for bottled water, a *billion* dollar industry.

The sources of water contamination are myriad. The list includes industrial waste, the underground disposal of extremely hazardous toxins through injection wells, and leaking underground fuel tanks. Then there's the agricultural runoff of pesticides, the toxic runoff from streets and rooftops of chemicals used in paving and building materials, and the radioactive contamination of radium, a by-product of the decay of uranium, used in nuclear power plants.

One of the most talked about contaminants in our drinking water is chlorine, a necessary disinfectant used to kill harmful, disease-causing bacteria. Unfortunately, chlorine combines easily with other chemicals and naturally occurring organic material to form many carcinogenic substances. An example of this is *trihalomethanes* (THMs), which are associated with rectal, bladder and pancreatic cancers, and may cause

The Truth About Your Drinking Water—CONTINUED

damage to the nervous system. Chlorine has also been linked to heart attacks, strokes, premature senility and sexual impotency. When you think about it, the purpose of chlorine is to kill living organisms; as far as I know we are all living organisms! Even in small amounts, taken daily this poison builds up in our systems and causes harm.

There is a simple test kit you can buy from any pool or spa store to check the amount of chlorine in your water. You squirt a few drops of a substance called *orthotolidene* (OTO) into the water, and it turns the water yellow to indicate the level of chlorine. You compare the tested water to the color bar, and if the water is too yellow, it's considered unsafe to swim in. Yet many times, if you use this test on your tap water, you'll find it at the top of the chart — in other words, not safe to swim in, let alone drink! Now, we wouldn't go to our swimming pool and dip out some water to drink or cook our food in, would we? But many people are doing the equivalent of that without realizing it.

Lead is another major contaminant. Today one in nine children under the age of six is said to have unacceptably high blood levels. I don't know about you, but none of the children I know sit around eating paint chips off walls — the lead is in the drinking water, and foods and beverages prepared with water. According to the Department of Health and Human Services, lead is the number one environmental threat to children. The EPA has actually concluded that there is no "safe" exposure to lead. It causes learning disabilities in children, delays normal physical and mental development in babies and toddlers, is linked to *hypertension* (high blood pressure) in adults, and can cause damage to the nervous system, kidneys and reproductive system. Lead is implicated in causing leukemia as well.

Unfortunately, I must alarm you further and mention that in addition to chemical toxins in our water such as chlorine, lead, pesticides, etc., we also need to be concerned about microbiological threats. Traditional water purification measures are ineffective against many waterborne diseases, especially some virulent newcomers. The *Centers for Disease Control* (CDC) has actually issued several warnings in recent years to people who are aged or suffering from immune deficiency disorders not to drink tap water, because their bodies are not strong enough to fight off water-borne infections.

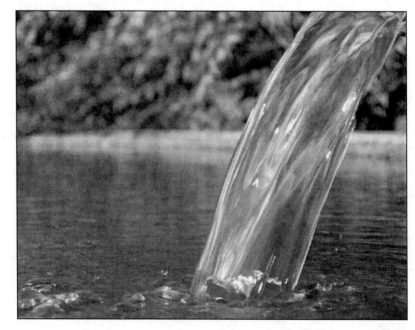

In 1993 in Milwaukee there was an outbreak of *cryptosporidium* that made thousands ill. *Giardia* is another common threat; although it won't kill you, it can make you quite uncomfortable, causing nausea, diarrhea and other digestive disorders. In 1991 and 1992, seventeen states reported outbreaks of

The Truth About Your Drinking Water—CONTINUED

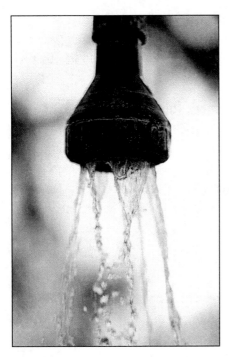

disease associated with drinking water, affecting over 17,000 people. But the CDC believes that outbreaks of waterborne disease are probably under-recognized and under-reported, in part because reporting outbreaks is voluntary in the United States.

One last thing to mention, which is very important, is that even if you are drinking clean water (bottled from some pristine spring in the mountains or filtered with a state-of-the-art filtration system), if you are showering in chlorinated water you still face health risks. When water is heated up and becomes steam in the shower, the chemicals evaporate out and are inhaled. The amount of chlorine absorbed by your body in just a ten minute shower is the equivalent to your drinking two gallons of tap water! According to the *American Journal of Public Health:*

> *"Skin absorption of contaminants has been underestimated and ingestion may not constitute the sole or even primary route of exposure."*

Since I began researching this issue, I have been completely shocked and horrified to discover all that I just detailed. (And, of course, there's much more.) The first step is in raising awareness on the issue. I would recommend that everyone explore this subject and re-evaluate what they are putting into their bodies and the bodies of their children. Luckily, there are products on the market that offer solutions, and in some areas the government is actually requiring all new homes to be built with a water filtration system from the start.

You're Not Sick, You're Thirsty!
Not drinking enough water can be the cause of many different health problems

by F. Batmanghelidj, M.D.

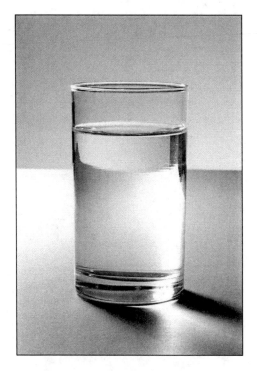

The human body is about 75% water and 25% solid matter. The brain is said to be 85% water and is extremely sensitive to any dehydration or depletion of its water content. It is water that regulates all the functions of the body, including the action of all the solids that water carries around.

There has been a groundbreaking medical breakthrough that is very significant. Simply put, it is the "new scientific understanding" that chronic unintentional dehydration can manifest itself in many ways — as many ways as we in medicine have invented diseases. Tragically, this medical breakthrough is not reaching the public through the health maintenance systems.

It is estimated that more than 110 million people in America are prone to suffer from various pains; in some cases with crippling intensity. "Pain of dehydration" afflicts Americans in various ways not usually associated with dehydration. They are:

Arthritis: The largest sector of our society manifests their chronic unintentional dehydration in the form of arthritic pains.

Heartburn: Reflecting dehydration, heartburn destroys many a night's rest or a day's peace of mind for millions of people.

Back Pain: This devastating pain is a periodic yearly affliction for over 30 million people.

Migraines: The debilitating pain of migraine headaches devastates the lives many.

Colitis: This pain is associated with constipation and digestion and affects a large sector of our society

Fibromyalgia: The pain felt in the muscles and joints all over the body is a crippling problem.

Angina: Since *angina* (chest pain) is an ominous sign of impending heart attacks and possible death, it is the most feared of all body pains.

You're Not Sick, You're Thirsty! Not drinking enough water can be the cause of many different health problems—CONTINUED

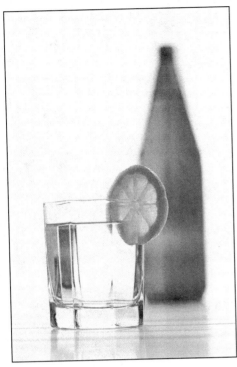

To relieve these devastating pains, a variety of pain medications have been produced and prescribed by doctors who never realized the physiologic significance of why the human body possesses a pain alarm system at all, and what is the common factor and trigger mechanism for these pains. Since these pains are felt in different locations, obviously they meant different diseases, or so it seemed! Because pain research has until now focused entirely on its solid composition, the common factor of water shortage in the interior of the body had not been apparent.

The new scientific understanding since 1987 is that localized or regional dehydration is the primary common factor and pain-producing problem of the human body. It becomes established when there is persistent regional water shortage, including in the interior of the pain-sensing nerve cells in the human body. This is the common factor to all body pains. In drought management mode, and when there is not enough "fresh water" to go around and wash out the toxic by-products of metabolism from the areas that are engaged in continuous activity, the nerve endings in those areas sense the increased toxicity, sound the alarm of pain and force the person to stop doing whatever is increasing toxic waste production — hence the loss of function in painful areas.

For example, when the heart muscle itself is short of "fresh water" and yet has to beat faster and forcefully to cope with any strenuous physical undertaking, pain is produced. In that instance, pain means thirst for "fresh water," even if it is believed that the blood flow to the heart muscle is reduced because of narrowing of its blood vessels. Interestingly, even cholesterol plaque formations in the heart arteries are caused by the same dehydration.

In treatment of chronic pains of the body, simple water has natural medicinal effects far superior to any pain medication. Pain medications shut down the crisis calls of the body for water, but do not correct the "fresh water" shortage in the interior of the body. On the other hand, water intake corrects the basic pain-producing drought and saves the body from further danger.

Women's Eating Habits & Health Concerns: Nutritional Support for Balancing Weight, Mood and Menopause

by Edward Bauman, M.Ed., Ph.D.

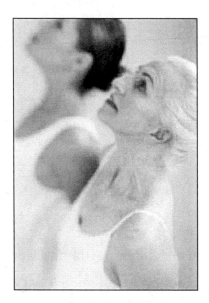

Despite the fact that two out of three health care dollars are spent on women, they are still not being listened to. Women's wisdom is generally ignored by mainstream health practitioners. Women's body knowledge is dismissed as "neurotic," "hypochondriac," or "hysterical." The medical establishment is so dominated by men's thinking and male physiology that women's different hormonal make-up and health needs are rarely in the conscious awareness of physicians.[1]

For all of us, neuro-hormonal balance is the key to well-being. Diet, exercise, environment, and attitude are modulators of hormonal health. What we eat, therefore, has a profound influence on how we act and feel now and later in life,[2] yet little attention has been paid to the negative effects of poor eating habits and other lifestyle choices on women's hormonal health.

Regardless of gender, race, age, and one's likes or dislikes, all human beings have three essential activities in common — movement, breathing, and eating.[3] How many busy people are watching what they eat, how they move, and if their breathing is shallow or deep? Life in the fast lane creates stress, disrupts awareness, and diverts our attention from living *well*.

This article discusses the impact of diet, lifestyle, and environment on health issues that concern all women and preoccupy many: finding balance with weight, mood, and menopause.

Diet Destruction

Much has been written about the stereotypes that have been inflicted on women in our culture. Women are expected to be thin, athletic, and attractive, while working long hours both inside and outside the home and coping with a myriad of stressors. They are constantly fed mixed-messages about what to eat, drink, smoke, and consume as medicine, hormones, cosmetics, and nutrients.

According to Bob Schwartz in his book *Diets Still Don't Work*,[4] there have been as many as 26,000 different diets "sold" over the years. Many women have tried, and continue to try, the latest fad diet, which is seldom based on sound nutritional science, rejuvenation principles, or health-building practices. Dieters are trapped in a cycle of:

▶ Setting unrealistic goals;

▶ Eating less food;

▶ Destabilizing blood sugar;

▶ Binging and starving;

▶ Down-regulating metabolism;

▶ Up-regulating fat storage;

▶ Inducing stress and toxicity;

▶ Triggering neuro-hormonal compensations; and

▶ Fighting depression and fatigue.

Women's Eating Habits & Health Concerns: Nutritional Support for Balancing Weight, Mood and Menopause—CONTINUED

The problems of weight mismanagement, mood swings, and hormone imbalance worsen the longer a women is eating too little nutrient-dense food and too much non-nutritive food. It is all too common for women to "yo-yo" between:

- ► High-protein, low-carbohydrate diets;
- ► High-carbohydrate, low-protein diets;
- ► No-fat or lowfat diets;
- ► Low-calorie fasting diets; and
- ► Caffeinated, thermogenic diet pills and powders

Food Models, Old and New

The science of nutrition is less than 50 years old. Currently, we are experiencing a renaissance in understanding the biochemical needs of individuals across a life span. Much clinical research has been undertaken to investigate the role of single nutrients on disease prevention and management, while too little attention has been put on studying what supports health, longevity, and hormone balance.

I have developed a whole foods model called *Eating For Health*™ that is plant-based, local, seasonal, and organic. It serves as a dramatic alternative to the U.S. Department of Agriculture's *Four Food Groups*[5] that most Americans were raised on, and to the federal government's 1992 Food Pyramid that is taught in schools and considered by many people to represent a well-balanced diet.

One must question why women who were raised on conventional American food such as these two official systems recommend commonly fight battles with weight, mood, and hormones. Might there be something lacking in our food, or something added to our food, that is disturbing our metabolism?

Diets recommended by the USDA and major food manufacturers have done an excellent job of selling the American public on the merits of post-World War II food commodities. The fresh-from-the-farm food our grandparents raised and ate has been largely supplanted by supermarket, restaurant, and convenience foods that are packaged, processed, and prepared for rapid heating and eating. There has been little awareness, until recently, of the quality and health impacts of food saturated with commercial fertilizers, herbicides, pesticides, and fungicides; chlorinated and fluoridated water; and genetically modified organisms.

We ignore these things at our peril, for as the food of a nation is compromised, so too is its vitality and health.

Food Sensitivities

Sensitivity to the following ingredients in common foods may cause women to suffer multiple problems that they and their physicians do not associate with diet:

- ► Additives;
- ► Coloring agents;
- ► Natural and artificial flavors;
- ► Artificial sweeteners; and
- ► Stabilizers and preservatives.

Women's Eating Habits & Health Concerns: Nutritional Support for Balancing Weight, Mood and Menopause—CONTINUED

When women consume these "reactive" foods, they may experience such symptoms as:

▶ Tissue swelling;

▶ Abdominal bloating;

▶ Metabolic disturbances;

▶ Weight gain; and

▶ Mood disorders.

An estimated 80 to 90% of all significantly overweight people suffer from these reactions and can lose weight if the condition is corrected.[6] Food reactions are the single most common cause of the cravings that derail diets. These cravings, which are far harder to resist than mere hunger, are similar to the physical urges experienced by alcoholics or cigarette smokers. A *Food Reaction/Health Disturbance Cycle*[7] (see the next page) begins in infancy with an inappropriate diet of commercial "formula" and refined foods. Food reactions increase the total load on young and growing women's immune systems throughout their life spans.

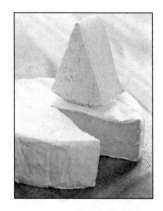

The Sensitive Seven: Most Common Reactive Foods

▶ Dairy products

▶ Wheat products

▶ Corn

▶ Sugar

▶ Soy

▶ Eggs

▶ Peanuts

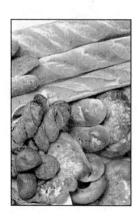

Risk Factors that Cause Food Reactions

According to Elson Haas, MD, the primary cause of food reactions is incomplete digestion. Food that is not well digested can enter our system as macromolecules. These remnants of poor digestion are perceived as antigens, or foreign substances that trigger immune reactions, fatigue, weight gain, mood disorders, congestion, and fat gain. Haas identifies several factors that contribute to poor digestion[7]:

Risk Factor 1:

Eating too narrow a range of foods. The average American gets about 75% of daily calories from as few as 10 different foods. Furthermore, the most common reactive foods are the most frequently consumed foods.

Risk Factor 2:

Eating too many "fake" foods. Far too many synthetic products have entered the food system. Diet foods, such as artificial sugars (*Nutrasweet*®) and fake fat (*Olestra*) are not properly metabolized into usable energy. Low-calorie foods are loaded with starches, gums, food additives, colorings, and preservatives.

Women's Eating Habits & Health Concerns: Nutritional Support for Balancing Weight, Mood and Menopause—CONTINUED

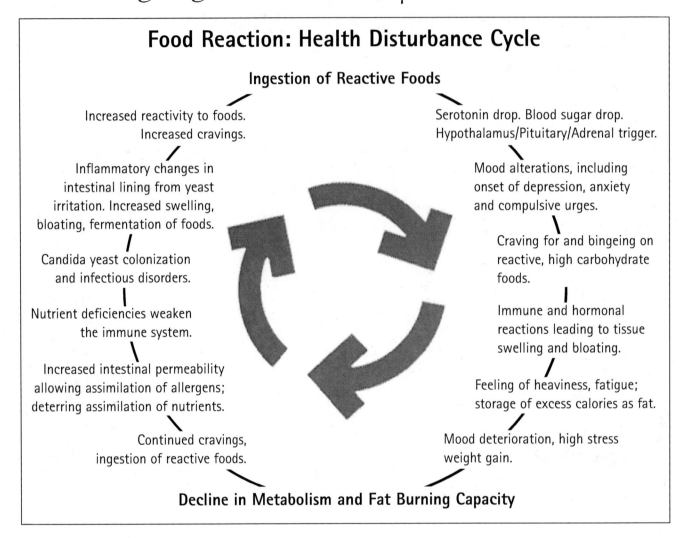

Food Reaction: Health Disturbance Cycle

Ingestion of Reactive Foods

Increased reactivity to foods.
Increased cravings.

Inflammatory changes in intestinal lining from yeast irritation. Increased swelling, bloating, fermentation of foods.

Candida yeast colonization and infectious disorders.

Nutrient deficiencies weaken the immune system.

Increased intestinal permeability allowing assimilation of allergens; deterring assimilation of nutrients.

Continued cravings, ingestion of reactive foods.

Serotonin drop. Blood sugar drop. Hypothalamus/Pituitary/Adrenal trigger.

Mood alterations, including onset of depression, anxiety and compulsive urges.

Craving for and bingeing on reactive, high carbohydrate foods.

Immune and hormonal reactions leading to tissue swelling and bloating.

Feeling of heaviness, fatigue; storage of excess calories as fat.

Mood deterioration, high stress weight gain.

Decline in Metabolism and Fat Burning Capacity

Risk Factor 3:

Having digestive enzyme deficiencies. Genetics, stress, and poor diet weaken our digestive capacity as we age. Taking over-the-counter antacids and prescription medications for digestive distress inhibits gastric output, bile, and pancreatic secretions. Our digestive enzymes and hormones depend upon a daily supply of amino acids, minerals, and B-complex vitamins to function optimally.

Risk Factor 4:

Eating food that is too refined. Excessive food processing robs foods of fiber and nutrients. Refined carbohydrates rapidly enter the blood stream, raising insulin levels. Insulin resistance is the body's way of saying "no thanks" to nutrient-deficient, calorie-rich blood. High blood sugar is converted to triglycerides and stored as body fat, unless a person is physically or metabolically active.

Women's Eating Habits & Health Concerns: Nutritional Support for Balancing Weight, Mood and Menopause—CONTINUED

Risk Factor 5:

Creating intestinal problems. Years of poor eating habits and choices give rise to a condition called dysbiosis, or poor intestinal ecology. The chronic ingestion of reactive foods taken with coffee, soft drinks, alcohol, and chemical additives inflame the membranes of the small intestine, causing a hyper-permeability, or *Leaky Gut Syndrome* (LGS). GI inflammation allows the passage of undigested food particles into the blood stream. Adding further insult to injury is an overgrowth of pathogenic bacteria or yeast that proliferates when a woman regularly ingests substances that have adverse effects on intestinal health such as:

- ▶ Antibiotics;
- ▶ Birth control pills;
- ▶ Steroid drugs;
- ▶ Refined carbohydrates;
- ▶ Yeasted foods such as bread, beer, wine, mushrooms; or
- ▶ Insufficient whole foods with fiber, flora, and fluids intact.

Candida overgrowth (*candidiasis*) is a major cause of bloating and stomach distension due to chronic gas and inflammation. Candida contributes to foggy thinking, toxemia, and low energy. Dysbiosis can be corrected by eating a protein and vegetable diet, along with essential fatty acids, and taking antifungal herbs and spices, such as garlic, Pau D'Arco, uva ursi, grapefruit seed extract, and caprylic and undecylenic acids.

Risk Factor 6:

Eating too much at once. Overeating overwhelms the digestive system. Craving reactive foods further compounds compulsive overeating. With allergic addiction, one feels better when a reactive food is consumed, as it generates an immediate hyper-metabolic reaction. When this wears off, the person experiences a hypo-metabolic withdrawal and, often, depression. Upon eating an addictive food, the person feels better for a little while, and then the problems return. This cycle is debilitating and results in numerous antigens and calories.

Risk Factor 7:

Being under too much stress. Stress inhibits digestion, growth, and cellular repair. The stress hormones, adrenaline and cortisol, draw blood away from the organs of digestion and feed the nerves, muscles, heart, and brain. With stress, too little blood that is rich in amino and fatty acids, vitamins, and minerals is available to nourish the thyroid, pancreas, and liver, thus compromising digestion, assimilation, and detoxification.

Risk Factor 8:

Not taking enough time to eat. Eating is a great pleasure and reward for most of us. Nevertheless, meals are often skipped, rushed, eaten on the run or in the car, and consumed at odd hours of the day and night. It takes very little to interrupt our digestion — noise, arguments, television, work, and family needs

Women's Eating Habits & Health Concerns: Nutritional Support for Balancing Weight, Mood and Menopause—CONTINUED

are common distractions. Making a commitment to eat in peace is an important first step to improving digestion and restoring balance to the neuro-endocrine system.

Vegetables without Vitamins

Nutritionist Alex Jack compared the US Department of Agriculture food tables from 1963 to 2000.[8] To his (and our) dismay, he found that the nutrient value of over a dozen fruits and vegetables has dropped precipitously. For example:

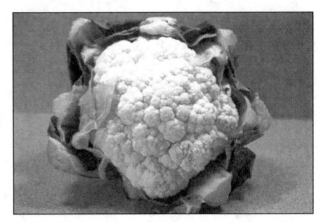

▶ Broccoli's calcium and Vitamin A content has dropped by 50%;

▶ Collard greens — long thought to be a staple of vitamins and minerals — dropped per serving from 6500 IUs of Vitamin A to 3800 IUs. Their potassium per serving has dropped from 400mg to 170mg. Magnesium content has fallen from 57mg to 9mg per serving; and

▶ Cauliflower has lost almost half its Vitamin C, along with its thiamin and riboflavin.

To make matters worse, Harry Balzer, Vice President of NPD Group,[9] a firm that gathers information on the eating habits of Americans, says that the preferred American meal is a one-dish, already prepared concoction. Unless a vegetable can be squirted out of a bottle (ketchup), it's frequently missing from our meals. Within the last 15 years, the percentage of all dinners including just one vegetable other than salad or potatoes dropped 10 to 41%. Balzar states that pizza is our favorite meal. Our other most popular foods include bread, doughnuts, pasta, cheese, beef, and milk. Without fortified cereal — which itself can't be considered a whole, natural food — Americans would not come close to meeting the *Recommended Daily Allowances* (RDA) for nutrients.[9]

According to one study, less than one-third of Americans get the minimum five servings of fruits and vegetables a day.[10] Only about 10% of Americans buy healthy groceries. The other 90% rely on ketchup, chips, onions, fat-free snacks, hot dogs, ice cream, cheese, and *Sweet Tarts*™ as their sources of nutrition.[9]

In the world of produce, nutritional content is generally considered much less important than things like appearance and big yield. Commercial growers view food as a product in the same way that running shoes are a product. In their eyes, looks are more important than substance.[5]

Scientists from *Doctor's Data Lab* tested whether foods labeled "organic" had greater nutritive concentrations. A comparison of the mineral levels of supermarket vs. organic produce from the Chicago, Illinois area[11] looked at apples, pears, potatoes, corn, wheat berries, and flour and found that the organic foods had, on average, twice the elemental mineral concentrations on a fresh weight basis as commercial foods

Women's Eating Habits & Health Concerns: Nutritional Support for Balancing Weight, Mood and Menopause—CONTINUED

of comparable size and weight. Equally important, toxic elements like aluminum, cadmium, lead, and mercury were found to be less prevalent in organic foods, on average, than in the supermarket foods tested.

Dietary Supplements

Dietary supplements have proven their worth in scientific studies conducted worldwide. Cancer, heart disease, bone loss, blood sugar disorders, stroke, and macular degeneration have been shown to be prevented, delayed, or ameliorated by the right combination of nutrients given in supplemental form.

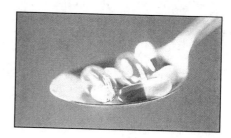

For example, nurses who took multi-vitamins containing folic acid for fifteen years slashed their risk of colon cancer by 75%. Folate from food did not work as well. No one knows why, although bioavailability problems are suspected. It is estimated that 90% of the population gets less folate per day than is necessary for health, a mere 400 micrograms.[12]

In the same nurses' study, women who took multi-vitamins containing Vitamin B6 reduced their risk of heart disease by 30%. The more B6 they took the lower the risk. Vitamin B6, along with magnesium, zinc, and Vitamin E are beneficial in hormone synthesis and regulation. With the nutrient content of food decreasing and the eating habits of many women less than optimal, taking high-quality nutritional supplements makes good health sense.

The following quoted studies in peer-reviewed journals demonstrate the associations between poor nutrition and premature illness and between improved nutrition and increased health and longevity:

"90% of women and 71% of men get less than the RDA for Vitamin B6."

Kant, AK et. al.[13]

"American children have inadequate levels of Vitamin E."

Bendich, A[14]

"The area of China with the lowest micronutrient intake has the highest rate of cancer. Vitamin E, selenium and beta-carotene lowers the rate."

Blot, WJ[15]

The following female eating habits and choices are likely contributors to the growing problems many women experience related to managing weight, mood, and menopause:

▶ Food quality is diminishing in the U.S. due to soil depletion and conventional farming practices;

▶ Women are routinely not taking the time to eat nutrient-rich meals;

▶ Food and environmental sensitivities are triggering many unpleasant reactions; and

▶ Many women are deficient in the nutrients necessary to sustain health and prevent disease.

Women's Eating Habits & Health Concerns: Nutritional Support for Balancing Weight, Mood and Menopause—CONTINUED

The longer poor eating habits persist, the deeper the depletion of nutritional reserves and digestive factors. The rising incidence of women's health concerns correlate with long-term poor nutrition, chronic stress, and neuro-hormonal depletion.

How to Build Health by Improving Diet and Nutrition

Many women experience frustration when confronted with symptoms of poor health such as weight gain, mood swings, and menopausal discomforts. They have never learned or practiced a health-building diet, daily exercise, and positive inner life. Under stress, a woman may slip from bad to worse in terms of food habits and choices.

The solution is making more conscious choices, reducing or eliminating foods on the following list of *Dietary Offenders* that diminish a woman's diet and health, and gradually adding in healthy foods from the list of *Dietary Rejuvenators* (see next page).

Nutrition can be likened to a bank account. Withdrawals come from eating *Dietary Offenders* that deplete nutritional reserves. Deposits come from eating *Dietary Rejuvenators,* which increase nutritional reserves. The interest you earn is the strength and vitality that comes with smart investing.

To create or restore adequate biochemical support for the neuro-hormonal system, daily ingestion of many of the following *Dietary Rejuvenators* is advised. Ingesting any of the Dietary Offenders will either displace or compete with the absorption of vital nutrients.

Ten Worst Dietary Offenders

Excessive (>1 serving/week) intake of any of these is not healthy:

- ▶ Fried foods:
  - French fries
  - Fried fish
  - Fried chicken
  - Onion rings or any other deep-fried snacks
- ▶ Salty snack foods:
  - Chips
  - Pretzels
  - Peanuts
- ▶ Fat-free or sugar-free desserts:
  - Frozen yogurt
  - Cookies

- ▶ Sugar/fat or flour confections:
  - Cookies
  - Candy
  - Ice cream
- ▶ Fast food burgers
- ▶ Meat-topped pizza
- ▶ Regular or diet sodas
- ▶ Tap water, coffee drinks, and alcohol
- ▶ Large meals at night
- ▶ Overeating anytime, anywhere, with anyone

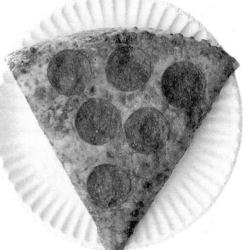

Women's Eating Habits & Health Concerns: Nutritional Support for Balancing Weight, Mood and Menopause—CONTINUED

Ten Best Dietary Rejuvenators

Eat as many foods as possible each day from these lists to provide essential nutrients for growth and repair.

▶ Protein foods:
- Lamb
- Poultry
- Fish
- Eggs
- Legumes
- Algae

▶ Essential fatty acid foods:
- Fish
- Flax
- Nuts and seeds

▶ Salad and cooking oils:
- Olive
- Avocado
- Coconut
- Ghee
- Butter

▶ Cultured dairy:
- Yogurt
- Kefir
- Buttermilk
- Feta cheese
- Blue cheese

▶ Non-glutenous grains:
- Rice
- Millet
- Quinoa
- Corn
- Buckwheat

▶ Soy foods:
- Miso
- Tamari
- Tempeh
- Tofu
- Yogurt
- Edamame
- Milk

▶ Cruciferous vegetables:
- Cabbage
- Broccoli
- Brussels sprouts
- Cauliflower

▶ Leafy greens:
- Kale
- Collards
- Chard
- Spinach
- Arugula
- Dark leaf lettuce

▶ Seasonal fruits:
- Citrus
- Apples
- Grapes
- Pears
- Figs
- Dates
- Prunes
- Apricots

▶ Culinary herbs and spices:
- Basil
- Oregano
- Thyme
- Garlic
- Ginger
- Turmeric

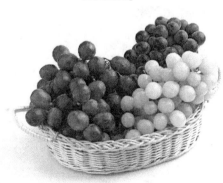

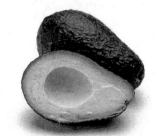

Women's Eating Habits & Health Concerns: Nutritional Support for Balancing Weight, Mood and Menopause—CONTINUED

Finally... A Neuro-Hormonal Diet Plan

A whole food, plant-based, diversified *Eating For Health*™ food plan is remarkably easy to shop for, eat, and store for quick, easy, and healthy future meals. Buy organic varieties and those free of hormones, antibiotics, chemicals, and genetically modified organisms whenever possible.

Build a meal plan that has:

- ▶ 25% calories from proteins;
- ▶ 25% calories from fats; and
- ▶ 50% calories from complex carbohydrates.

This ratio of high-quality, moderate-quantity whole foods can replenish the nutrient depletions responsible for creating metabolic imbalances and their unwanted symptoms of weight gain, mood swings, and hormonal symptoms. To construct a *Rejuvenating Diet Plan*, the following combinations and quantities are advised. For fine-tuning, it is advisable to consult with a qualified nutrition professional.

Breakfast, Snack or Dessert

- ▶ 1 serving dairy (6-8 oz. fermented cow, goat, or soy dairy)
- ▶ 0-1 serving fat (1 Tbsp. seeds or nuts)
- ▶ 2 servings fruit (a serving is 1 piece of whole fruit, 1/2 cup stewed or pureed fruit, OR 1/2 cup dried fruit)

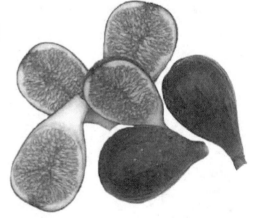

Lunch or Dinner

- ▶ 1 serving protein (2-3 oz. animal protein, 1 egg, or 4 oz. cooked legumes)
- ▶ 1 serving fat (1 tsp. oil or 1 Tbsp. seeds or nuts)
- ▶ 0-1 serving grains or starch (1/2 cup cooked cereal, 2/3 cup cooked pasta, 1 medium potato or yam, 1 cup baked winter squash, OR 1 slice of whole grain bread)
- ▶ 1-2 servings vegetables (a serving is 1 cup leafy greens OR 1/2 cup raw or steamed vegetables)

Factors of age, activity level, health condition, access to foods, and digestibility can be discussed with a professional nutrition consultant to insure a smooth dietary transition.

Healthy foods taste wonderful and are very satisfying. The key to improved nutrition is to make every bite count — to not ingest empty calories and artificial ingredients. For an attitudinal boost, adopt this *Eating For Health*™ affirmation, repeating it to yourself many times throughout the day:

"I always eat the freshest, most nutritious foods available."

Women's Eating Habits & Health Concerns: Nutritional Support for Balancing Weight, Mood and Menopause—CONTINUED

Vitality Shakes

A *Vitality Shake* is another quick and nourishing meal for breakfast, snack, or dessert. Here is how to prepare it. Combine the following ingredients in a blender and puree:

- ▶ 1 serving of fermented milk (yogurt or kefir)
- ▶ 1 serving of seeds or nuts
- ▶ 2 servings of seasonal fresh or dried fruit

Booster Food additions to the shake can include:

- ▶ 1 tsp.–1 Tbsp. green powder (Spirulina, chlorella, wheatgrass, and/or barley grass)
- ▶ 1 tsp.–2 Tbsp. whey or soy protein powder
- ▶ 1–2 tsp. *ORAC Plus*® powder (fruit concentrate with herbal antioxidants)
- ▶ 1/2–1 tsp. Acidophilus
- ▶ 1 Tbsp. Lecithin
- ▶ 1/2–1 tsp. l-Glutamine (a brain/liver/gut-friendly amino acid)
- ▶ 1/2–1 tsp. buffered Vitamin C powder

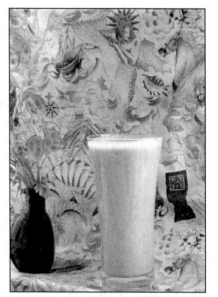

Applying Clinical Nutrition Research to Women's Health Concerns

In an integrative model, four variables should be considered in applying clinical research to women's health concerns:

- ▶ The uniqueness of the life experience of the woman seeking help;
- ▶ The interrelationship of all her presenting concerns;
- ▶ Peer-reviewed literature demonstrating the risks and benefits of various diet or nutritional interventions; and
- ▶ The sensitivity, time, and skill of the practitioner in explaining to the woman how her body has come to be in this state and teaching her, in several lessons, what she can do to improve and recover her health.

The combination of relevant information, personal support, and targeted nutrition improves the likelihood that a woman will commit to and follow through on making a change in her diet and assume the cost and effort of taking additional nutritional supplements.

Whenever a nutrient is deemed by the literature to be helpful in supporting a tissue or system that is in sub-optimal condition in an individual woman, advising her on dietary sources for the nutrient is the first means to be considered. If the dosage level indicated by the literature is greater than can be gained by eating food, then a dietary supplement may be recommended, including specific instructions for and monitoring of dose, duration, and interaction with other foods, beverages, herbs, nutrients, or medications.

Women's Eating Habits & Health Concerns: Nutritional Support for Balancing Weight, Mood and Menopause—CONTINUED

CONCLUSION

This article has considered the relationship between women's dietary habits and their health concerns, notably difficulties in balancing weight, mood, and menopausal symptoms across the lifespan. I have suggested that such symptoms result from a longstanding consumption of the modern refined and processed diet, and that diet-induced nutrient deficiencies have compromised many women's neuro-hormonal systems.

A common response to weight, mood, and menopausal challenges is to use over-the-counter, prescription medications or hormone replacement therapy, which are likely to further exacerbate the problems. The wide range of dietary and nutrient factors discussed in this article can address areas of weakness and provide optimal nutrition for overworked and underfed organs, glands, and tissues, significantly boosting a woman's health and sense of wellness at any age.

REFERENCES

1. Vliet, E. *Screaming To Be Heard.* M. Evans and Company. New York. 2001.
2. Bauman, 2001
3. Bland, J. *Genetic Nutritioneering.* Keats Publishing. Los Angeles. 1999.
4. Schwartz, B. *Diets Still Don't Work.* Breakthru Publishing. Houston. 1990.
5. USDA Food Tables. www.usda.gov. 2000.
6. Haas, E. *The False Fat Diet.* Ballentine Books. New York. 2000.
7. Haas, R. *Eat to Win for Permanent Weight Loss.* Harmony Books. New York. 2000.
8. Staff, *Vegetables Without Vitamins.* Life Extension Magazine (www.lef.org), 28-33. March, 2001.
9. NPD Group, Inc. "Highlights from the 15th Annual Report on Eating Patterns in America." www.npd.com. 2000.
10. Subar, AF et al. "Dietary sources of nutrients among U.S. adults, 1989-91." *J AM Diet Association.* 98:37-47. 1998.
11. Smith, BL. "Organic Foods vs. Supermarket Foods: Elemental Levels." *J Applied Nutrition* Vol. 43(1) 35-9. 1993.
12. Giovanucci, E et al. "Multivitamin use, folate and colon cancer in women in the nurses' health study." *Annals of Internal Medicine.* 129:517-24. 1998.
13. Kant, AK et al. "Dietary Vitamin B-6 Intake and food sources in the U.S. population." *NHANES II,* 1976-80. 1990.
14. Bendich, A. "Vitamin E status of U.S. children." *J Am College of Nutrition.* 11:441-4. 1992.
15. Blot, WJ. "Vitamin/mineral supplementation and cancer risk: international chemoprevention trials." *Proc Soc Exp Biol Med.* 216: 291-6. 1997.
16. Werbach, M and Moss, J. *Textbook of Nutritional Medicine.* Third Line Press. Tarzana, CA. 1999.

BIBLIOGRAPHY

Abraham, G. "Management of the premenstrual tension syndrome: rationale for a nutritional approach." J Bland, Ed. 1986; *A Year in Nutritional Medicine.* New Canaan, CT. Keats Publishing. 1986.

Comstock, GW. "Serum retinol, beta-carotene, Vitamin E and selenium areas related to subsequent cancer of specific sites." *Am J Epidemiology.* 135:115-21. 1992.

Medford, L. *Why Can't I Lose Weight?* LDN Publishing. Tulsa, OK. 1999.

Peeke, P. *Fighting Fat after Forty.* Viking Press. New York. 2000.

Reversing Diabetes & Obesity Naturally: Nutritional Super Stars
by Ed Bauman, M.Ed., Ph.D., & Jodi Friedlander, M.S.

Diabetes: Bad Food and Sedentary Living in Action

"Diabesity" — diabetes combined with its evil twin, obesity — is epidemic in the United States. According to the *American Diabetes Association* (ADA), 20.8 million children and adults — 7.0% of the population — have diabetes, almost half of which is undiagnosed (American Diabetes Association, [ADA], 2006). In addition, they estimate that 54 million people have pre-diabetes. Most disturbing of all is that there are 176,500 cases of diabetes in the segment of the population that is under 20 years of age, with the overwhelming majority of these cases being Type 2, or *non-insulin dependent, diabetes mellitus* (NIDDM) (ADA, 2006). The occurrence among children has increased tenfold within the past 20 years (Olshansky et al., 2005).

Type 2 diabetes — formerly referred to as adult-onset diabetes — is the most prevalent, its occurrence increasing at an unprecedented rate. It can occur at any age and is regarded as a disease of metabolic imbalance brought about by diet and lifestyle choices, specifically too many refined carbohydrates, too few nutritious foods, and not enough exercise. There may, as well, be inherited factors that contribute to it, although this is not as clear as in Type 1 diabetes, which usually manifests in childhood through early adulthood and is an auto-immune disorder characterized by the inability of the beta cells of the pancreas to produce insulin (NDIC, 2006).

Type 2 diabetes typically begins with insulin resistance, when the body's cells can no longer "hear" insulin's signaling messages and cannot use this hormone efficiently to get glucose into the cells (NDIC, 2006). The pancreas will produce more and more insulin to keep up with the body's energy demands, but it will eventually lose its ability to produce enough in response to meals, at which point diabetes sets in (NDIC, 2006).

There is also a sub-set of NIDDM called *gestational diabetes*, which some women develop in the late stages of pregnancy. Though it generally resolves after the baby's birth, these women tend to be more likely to develop Type 2 diabetes later in life (NDIC, 2006). The consequences of Type 2 diabetes include kidney damage, poor circulation, and numbness in the feet, dangerous infections, and erectile dysfunction. More importantly, though, it often results in cardiovascular disease, which claims the lives of 80% of diabetics (Mateljian, 2006).

Want to Reverse Type 2 Diabetes? Commit to Be Well™

Numerous drugs are prescribed to control both Type 1and Type 2 diabetes, which can be life saving but often fail to heal underlying metabolic imbalances. The Bauman Nutrition approach provided by our dynamic "*Commit To Be Well*™ Six-Month Mentored Health Building Program" teaches people with health challenges such as diabetes a life-changing five-step process to regularly and joyfully:

Reversing Diabetes & Obesity Naturally: Nutritional Super Stars

—CONTINUED

1. Eat for health;

2. Identify and avoid food and environmental toxins;

3. Engage in a cross training exercise program;

4. Add key booster foods and supplemental nutrients; and

5. Practice positive coping when stressed.

Eating For Health™ — Not a Diet, but an Optimally Healthy Eating Decision

Eating For Health™ (Bauman, 2006) is a diversified, whole foods nutritional approach based on fresh, local, seasonal, colorful, whole foods that are as chemical free as possible, prepared with love and care, and eaten in a spirit of gratitude. Moderation is the meditation when eating for health.

By eating the best foods available in a consistent way at regular intervals, blood sugar needs are met and digestive function can be restored, with stress and toxins being minimized while peace and nutrients are maximized. This is in stark contrast to eating for convenience, which is typical of the meals and milieu of people with diabetes, who often snack throughout the day on processed snack foods and restaurant fare laced with artificial colors, flavors, preservatives, and stabilizers. Food addiction is an underlying problem for many people with blood sugar disorders. In response to the cellular survival signal for blood sugar, they crave such foods as diet sodas, coffee, dairy products, and refined carbohydrates like pastries and pasta. These addictive pseudo-foods provide a temporary lift and predictable fall, accompanied by aggravating withdrawal symptoms often diagnosed as anxiety, depression, attention deficits, and learning disorders. Neuro-degeneration and neuro-toxicity are the consequences of eating for energy rather than for health. Not a pretty picture!

The change to eating complex carbohydrates, quality proteins and fats, and health-promoting beverages alters the neuro-endocrine response from one of stress and inflammation to stability and regulated cellular nourishment and function. Our experience is that when people with diabetes understand the controllable variables in their

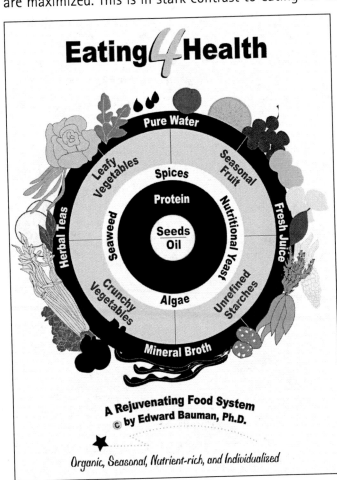

Eating 4 Health

Pure Water
Leafy Vegetables
Seasonal Fruit
Spices
Protein
Nutritional Yeast
Herbal Teas
Seaweed
Seeds Oil
Fresh Juice
Crunchy Vegetables
Algae
Unrefined Starches
Mineral Broth

A Rejuvenating Food System
© by Edward Bauman, Ph.D.

Organic, Seasonal, Nutrient-rich, and Individualized

Reversing Diabetes & Obesity Naturally: Nutritional Super Stars

—CONTINUED

condition — such as diet, exercise, attitude, and stress — they rise to the task of reversing a life time of poor eating and lifestyle habits and begin eating and acting for health.

Having a personal nutrition mentor in the *Commit To Be Well*™ (www.baumannutrition.com) program provides a balance of education, support, and encouragement that success is the reward for daily practice. In reversing an unhealthy diet and lifestyle, individuals can take great pride in watching their elevated blood sugar, insulin numbers, and scale weight fall as their natural vitality rises, marking the reversal of diabetes and obesity.

Feed Your Cells Nutritional Superstars

A growing body of scientific research has revealed that many single nutrients, herbs, and foods — the nutritional "superstars" — along with an *Eating For Health*™ diet provide substantial health benefits to slow and reverse diabetes and other inflammatory disorders, such as progressive neurological and cardio-vascular disease.

It should come as no surprise that, because diabetes can lead to circulatory and cardiovascular com-plications, a Mediterranean-type diet — which is highly recommended for heart health — also offers the most healthful options for a diabetic's diet. This regime, traditionally followed in Greece, Crete, southern France, and parts of Italy, is more a philosophy of eating than a rigid diet plan. It is comprised of the many foods indigenous to the region and can be adapted to reflect the offerings of any area of the world.

The main staples of Mediterranean cuisine include foods rich in mono- and Omega-3 poly-unsaturat-ed fats; lean proteins; and fruits, vegetables and whole grains that contain fiber and essential vitamins and minerals. In addition, scientific studies have demonstrated the usefulness of a number of culinary spices and medicinal herbs that may contribute to metabolic balance (Bruno, 2001; Kane, 1999; Mateljian, 2006; *National Library of Medicine* [NLM], 2005; Price, 2003). Some of these foods are discussed below.

While it is possible to supplement any diet with fatty acids, dietary fibers, and vitamins and minerals, due to the possibility of further damaging the metabolism with nutrient overdoses and imbalances, and because of known and as yet unknown synergistic effects, it is probably better to obtain as many of these nutrients as possible from foods.

Chili Peppers

Australian research recently published in the *American Journal of Clinical Nutrition* has shown that using chili peppers as a flavorful addition to foods, as opposed to the high doses one might find in supplements, allows the body to produce less insulin to transport glucose into cells. This prevents *hyperinsulinemia*, the condition of excessive blood levels and decreased hepatic clearance of insulin, associated with Type 2 diabetes (Ahuja et al., 2006). Positive results were obtained in this study when chilies were fed to subjects after a bland meal, but better results were obtained when the chilies were added to a background diet that

Reversing Diabetes & Obesity Naturally: Nutritional Super Stars

—CONTINUED

regularly included them as a spice, despite the fact that all the test diets (including the control diet) produced equivalent elevations in blood glucose. These beneficial effects on insulin improved as *body mass index* (BMI) increased, so that in very overweight people, the chili-containing meals had a greater effect. They not only lowered the amount of insulin required to decrease postprandial blood sugar levels, they also resulted in a lower *C-peptide/insulin quotient,* indicating that the liver's ability to clear insulin had improved (C-peptide is an indication of how much insulin is being released). The exact mechanism of action for this result is not completely understood, but the researchers believe that the lower glycemic response after the chili meals may have been due to reduced absorption and slower gastric emptying caused by the spice.

Cinnamon

The world's most-used spice, cinnamon has traditionally been used as a glucose-lowering agent. Little has been understood about how it works, though many scientists have recognized that it does. Recent research, though, done by the Agricultural Research Services division of the *United States Department of Agriculture* (USDA), has discovered the compound responsible for cinnamon's ability to enhance cells' insulin sensitivity (Anderson et al., 2000). These scientists, working with water extracts (not the oil extracts used as food additives), found that cinnamon's most active compound is a flavonoid called *methylhydroxy chalcone polymer* (MHCP), which was found to increase glucose metabolism 20-fold in in-vitro fat cells. In a blood platelet assay, MHCP prevented the formation of damaging oxygen radicals, and it was also found to reduce blood pressure in test rats before it produced its blood sugar results. This is a truly beneficial spice, and though the research was done with water extracts, using the ground spice would contain not only the active agents but also a little fiber, as well as the synergistic benefits that whole foods confer.

Cold Water Fish

Eating more wild-caught, cold-water fish such as salmon, cod, halibut, and herring provides some of the only food sources for the Omega-3 long-chain fatty acids, *eicosapentaenoic acid* (EPA) and *docosahexaenoic acid* (DHA). Omega-3 fats, including *alpha-linolenic acid* (ALA) from plant sources, have long been recognized as having beneficial effects on the cardiovascular system. They may also help prevent diabetes. Previous population studies done on overweight Eskimos who did not have diabetes or heart disease indicated that it was the Omega-3 fats portion of their traditional diet that provided protection from these conditions. In 2002, a small research study provided its overweight, insulin-resistant subjects with a moderate dose (1.8 gm) of DHA for three weeks (in Mercola, 2002). The results showed improvement in insulin sensitivity in 70% of its subjects, and in 50% of

Reversing Diabetes & Obesity Naturally: Nutritional Super Stars
—CONTINUED

those the change was statistically significant. In addition, EPA has been shown to stimulate secretion of the hormone *leptin,* which helps regulate food intake, metabolism, and body weight (Mateljian, 2006). These fish are also good sources of protein and contain many of the nutrients often lacking in diabetics: Vitamin B6, magnesium, zinc, and chromium (Mooradian et al., 1987). Other lean sources of protein also offer these other nutrients, and because animals are one of the best sources of *chromium* — an important factor in blood sugar regulation as part of the *Glucose Tolerance Factor* (GTF) molecule — they are highly recommended. Good sources include fish, but also turkey, chicken, and lean organic or grass-fed beef.

Olive Oil and Avocados

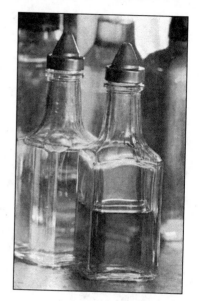

Eating avocados and replacing other dietary fats with olive oil may be one of the best, tastiest, and least known ways to manage blood sugar. Much attention is paid to the health benefits of supplemental fish oils, but recently published research has shown that very high doses can elevate blood glucose levels and decrease insulin sensitivity (Mostad et al., 2006). The authors of this study admit that the negative effects were minor and that, ingested in quantities found in the diet, no significant effects would be expected. But this study serves to illuminate how important it can be to supplement moderately, and that one set of nutrients cannot be expected to be a cure-all. Other research has clearly shown that the *monounsaturated fatty acids* (MUFA's), the main fatty acids in olive oil as well as avocados, may be an even more effective means of protecting the heart and preventing diabetes. Garg (1998), in a meta-analysis of studies done on the effects of MUFA's on subjects with diabetes mellitus, found that high-monounsaturated fat diets — up to 30% in the diet — consistently reduced fasting plasma triacylglycerol and VLDL-cholesterol concentrations by 19% and 22%, respectively. He also found improved glycemic control and modestly elevated HDL concentrations. Garg surmises that high-monounsaturated fat diets improve lipid profiles because they may "reduce the susceptibility of LDL particles to oxidation and thereby reduce their atherogenic potential." He is not sure why they improve glycemic control, but thinks it may simply be due to lower carbohydrate intake. Another study looked at research done comparing low-fat, high-carbohydrate diets to high-monounsaturated fat diets and found similar positive effects on glycemic control (Ros, 2003). Like Garg, Ros found improved lipid profiles in the MUFA diets and noted that low-fat diets "are associated with atherogenic, dense LDL particles, while normal, buoyant LDL predominates with high-fat diets irrespective of fatty acid composition". In addition to being one of the only food sources of MUFA's, avocados also provide B vitamins, magnesium, copper, and manganese in meaningful quantities.

Reversing Diabetes & Obesity Naturally: Nutritional Super Stars

—CONTINUED

Walnuts, Almonds, and Peanuts

While differing slightly in their specific nutrient profiles, these nuts (though peanuts are technically a *legume*) provide good sources of monounsaturated fats. Almonds and peanuts also contain Omega-6 fatty acids, one of the essential fats, meaning we need them in our diets because our bodies do not produce them naturally. Walnuts are a good source of the Omega-3 essential polyunsaturated fat, *alpha-linolenic acid* (ALA). The small amounts of saturated fat these nuts contain help ensure that the ALA will adequately be converted to the longer-chain fatty acids, EPA and DHA, in the body (Enig, 2000; p.107). In a study of 84,000 women in the Nurses' Health Study, eating nuts and peanut butter was inversely associated with Type 2 diabetes (Jiang, 2002). It is the researchers' belief that the unsaturated fats in nuts allow the body to utilize insulin more effectively and to regulate blood glucose. All nuts also contain small amounts of protein, loads of necessary fiber, and substantial quantities of many of the trace elements previously mentioned as often deficient in diabetics: zinc, magnesium, copper, and manganese (Mooradian et al., 1987).

Legumes and Whole Grains — Buckwheat and Oats

These are high-fiber carbohydrates, loaded with nutrients. Much research has been done over the years on food fibers and most, if not all, researchers are in agreement that diets high in soluble fiber are necessary to keep cholesterol and blood sugar levels under control (Fung et al., 2002; Hagander et al., 1988; Ou et al., 2001; Trowell, 1978). Whole grains appear to be particularly helpful, perhaps because of their relatively high levels of magnesium, which is associated with a lowered risk of Type 2 diabetes (Fung et al., 2002). Oats have often been touted for their ability to lower cholesterol levels, and they also help maintain glycemic control, but it looks as though barley, which contains four times the soluble fiber of oats, does a better job (Mateljian, 2006). Buckwheat, the grain often used in pancakes and soba noodles, has also come to the forefront of blood sugar control. A recent Canadian study found that extracts of buckwheat fed to Type 1 diabetic rats lowered glucose levels 12% to 19% (Przybylski, 2003). Previous findings led the study's researchers to believe that the active components in the buckwheat, bioflavonoids and inositol, rather than its fiber content, are the key factors. Rarely found in other foods, this substance is believed to either make cells more insulin sensitive or to act as an insulin mimic, though only preliminary research exists at this time (Przybylski, 2003). These two grains, along with brown rice, which is probably a more popular food, contain significant amounts of the B vitamins, copper, magnesium, and manganese, as well as moderate amounts of zinc. Beans and legumes are also good sources of the B vitamins, including B6, provide lean protein and fiber, and deliver much-needed magnesium.

Reversing Diabetes & Obesity Naturally: Nutritional Super Stars

—CONTINUED

Garlic

Both onions and garlic have been recognized as beneficial to health, especially heart health, but it looks like garlic may be the better food to control blood sugar levels. An Iranian study done in 2005 compared the glycemic-controlling properties of garlic, onions, and fenugreek, all recommended in Persian folklore medicine as beneficial in the treatment of diabetes (Jelodhar et al., 2005). A previous study, in 1996, found that fenugreek seed powder signifi-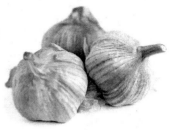
cantly lowered fasting blood glucose, improved glucose tolerance, and decreased insulin levels (Sharma et al., 1996). The spice also reduced urinary sugar excretion, and the researchers deemed it beneficial to diabetics. This more recent study, however, found that only garlic, in relation to the control group, caused any lowering of blood sugar, and that garlic's benefit was statistically significant (Jelodhar et al., 2005). This refutes the previous findings on fenugreek and also challenges claims concerning onion's lowering effect on blood sugar. Garlic's mechanism of action is unknown, but the researchers believe that plants may exert hypoglycemic effects due to: 1) their insulin-like substances, 2) stimulation of beta cells to produce more insulin, 3) high levels of fiber that slow carbohydrate digestion, or 4) their ability to regenerate pancreatic cells.

Bitter melon

A tropical fruit indigenous to Asia, East Africa, and South America, bitter melon can be purchased fresh in Asian markets or in extract form from natural foods stores. Several studies have shown that it can significantly lower both blood glucose and cholesterol levels (Price, 2003). Though researchers are not sure how bitter melon affects cholesterol, it is believed that its effect on blood sugar is due to an increase in the activity of *hexokinase* and *glucokinase*, enzymes that convert sugar into *glycogen*, which can be stored in the liver for future energy use (Price, 2003).

Eating For Health™: The rainbow provides the "pot of gold"

This list is by no means exhaustive. In fact, a varied whole foods diet, with or without these foods, will provide enormous benefits for preventing or reversing diabetes and maintaining overall health. In addition, please keep in mind that fruits and, especially, vegetables, contain some of the highest levels of vitamins and minerals — as well as large amounts of fiber — of any foods. They also provide a wide range of phytonutrients, health-promoting substances found only in plants. For all of these reasons, fruits and vegetables should be consumed several times daily.

Eating For Health™ is eating from the rainbow. Consuming a wide variety of colorful vegetables, fruits, and other foods on a regular basis provides the widest spectrum of health-giving nutrients and may help us all find our way to the "pot of gold" — our good health. In the process, we will leave behind our blood sugar irregularities and greatly reduce our risk of diabetes.

Reversing Diabetes & Obesity Naturally: Nutritional Super Stars

—CONTINUED

REFERENCES

Ahuja, Kiran DK; Robertson, Iain K; Geraghty, Dominic P; and Ball, Madeleine J. "Effects of Chili Consumption on Postprandial Glucose, Insulin, and Energy Metabolism." *American Journal of Clinical Nutrition,* online version. Jul 2006; 84: 63-69. Retrieved 11/1/06 from: http://www.ajcn.org/cgi/content/full/84/1/63#SEC4

Anderson, Richard A; Schmidt, Walter F; Broadhurst, C Leigh; and Polansky, Marilyn M. "Cinnamon Extracts Boost Insulin Sensitivity." July 2000. Cited in *United States Department of Agriculture's* (USDA) Agricultural Research Services website. Retrieved 11/08/06 from: http://www.ars.usda.gov/is/AR/archive/jul00/cinn0700.htm

Anonymous. "Total Prevalence of Diabetes and Pre-diabetes." 2006; *American Diabetic Association.* Retrieved 11/04/06: http://www.diabetes.org/diabetes-statistics/prevalence.jsp

Anonymous. "What Kind of Diabetes Do You Have? Your Guide to Diabetes: Type 1 and Type 2." *National Diabetes Information Clearinghouse* (NDIC), a service of National Institute of Diabetes and Digestive and Kidney Diseases, National Institutes of Health. April, 2006. Retrieved 11/06/06 from: http://diabetes.niddk.nih.gov/dm/pubs/type1and2/what.htm

Anonymous. *Type 2 Diabetes Mellitus. Description; Dietary Causes; Nutrient Needs; Nutrient Excesses; Recommended Diet.* 2006; The George Mateljan Foundation. Retrieved 11/02/06 from: http://whfoods.org/genpage.php?tname=disease&dbid=3

Balch, PA and Balch, JF. Diabetes. *Prescription for Nutritional Healing* (pp. 321-326). Penguin Putnam: New York. (2000).

Bruno, G. *Diabetes. Ailments and Natural Remedies.* (pp. 89-92). Fifty-ninth Street Bridge: New York. (2001).

Byrum, Allison. "Buckwheat May Be Beneficial for Managing Diabetes." American Chemical Society, November 18, 2003. Retrieved 11/05/06 from *Medical News Today* online: http://www.medicalnewstoday.com/medicalnews.php?newsid=4694

Enig, MG. *Know Your Fats.* Bethesda Press: Maryland (2000).

Fallon, S (with Enig, MG). *Nourishing Traditions, Revised Second Edition.* (pp. 22, 42-45, 617-620). New Trends: Washington, DC. (2001).

Fung, Teresa T; Hu, Frank B; Pereira, Mark A; Liu, Simin; Stampfer, Meir J; Colditz, Graham A; and Willett, Walter C. "Whole-grain Intake and the Risk of Type 2 Diabetes: A Prospective Study in Men." *American Journal of Clinical Nutrition.* September 2002; 76:3, 535-540. Online version. Retrieved 11/04/06 from: http://www.ajcn.org/cgi/content/full/76/3/535?maxtoshow=&HITS=10&hits=10&RESULTFORMAT=&fulltext=diabetes&searchid=1&FIRSTINDEX=30&sortspec=relevance&resourcetype=HWCIT

Gannon, Mary C; Nuttall, Frank Q; Saeed, Asad; Jordan, Kelly; and Hoover, Heidi. "An Increase In Dietary Protein Improves the Blood Glucose Response In Persons With Type 2 Diabetes." *American Journal of Clinical Nutrition.* October 2003; 78: 4, 734-741. Online version. Retrieved 11/04/06 from: http://www.ajcn.org/cgi/reprint/78/4/734?maxtoshow=&HITS=10&hits=10&RESULTFORMAT=&fulltext=diabetes&searchid=1&FIRSTINDEX=50&sortspec=relevance&resourcetype=HWCIT

Garg, A. "High-Monounsaturated-Fat Diets for Patients with Diabetes Mellitus: A Meta-analysis." *American Journal of Clinical Nutrition.* 1998; 67: 577S-582S, online version. Retrieved 11/04/06 from: http://www.ajcn.org/cgi/reprint/67/3/577S?maxtoshow=&HITS=10&hits=10&RESULTFORMAT=&fulltext=diabetes&searchid=1&FIRSTINDEX=60&sortspec=relevance&resourcetype=HWCIT

Hagander, B; Asp, NG; Efendic, S; Nilsson-Ehle, P; and Schersten, B. "Dietary Fiber Decreases Fasting Blood Glucose Levels and Plasma LDL Concentration in Non-Insulin-Dependent Diabetes Mellitus Patients." *American Journal of Clinical Nutrition.* May 1988; 47: 852 - 858. Retrieved 11/03/06 from: http://www.ajcn.org/cgi/content/abstract/47/5/852?maxtoshow=&HITS=10&hits=10&RESULTFORMAT=&fulltext=diabetes&searchid=1&FIRSTINDEX=70&sortspec=relevance&resourcetype=HWCIT

Higdon, Jane. Linus Pauling Institute. Oregon State University. Micronutrtient Information Center, online. 2006. Various articles on vitamins and minerals. Retrieved 11/06/06 from: http://lpi.oregonstate.edu/infocenter/

Reversing Diabetes & Obesity Naturally: Nutritional Super Stars
—CONTINUED

Jelodar Gholamali, A; Maleki, M; Motadayenm MH; Sirus, S. "Effect of Fenugreek, Onion and Garlic on Blood Glucose and Histopathology of Pancreas of Alloxan-induced Diabetic Rats." 2005. *Indian Journal of Medical Sciences.* 59:2. 64-69. Online version. Retrieved 11/08/06 from: http://www.indianjmedsci.org/article.asp?issn=0019-5359;year=2005; volume=59;issue=2;spage=64;epage=69;aulast=Jelodar

Jiang, Rui; Manson, JoAnn E; Stampfer, Meir J; Liu, Simin; Willett, Walter C; Hu, Frank B. "Nut and Peanut Butter Consumption and Risk of Type 2 Diabetes in Women." *Journal of the American Medical Association* (JAMA). 2002;288:2554-2560. Online abstract. Retrieved 11/07/06 from: http://jama.highwire.org/cgi/content/abstract/288/20/2554

Kane, Emily. "Diabetes: Adult-Onset Diabetes Mellitus (Type II)." 1999. Retrieved 11/05/06 from: http://www.dremilykane.com/ Adult Onset Diabetes

Mercola, J. "Fish Oil Helps Prevent Diabetes." From Annual Experimental Biology 2002 Conference New Orleans, LA April 21, 2002. Retrieved 11/07/06 from: http://www.mercola.com/2002/may/8/fish_oil.htm

Mooradian, AD and Morley, JE. "Micronutrient Status in Diabetes Mellitus." *American Journal of Clinical Nutrition,* 1987; 45: 877-895. Online version. Retrieved 11/04/06 from: http://www.ajcn.org/cgi/reprint/45/5/877?maxtoshow=&HITS=10&hits= 10&RESULTFORMAT=&fulltext=diabetes&searchid=1&FIRSTINDEX=0&sortspec=relevance&resourcetype=HWCIT

Mostad, Ingrid L; Bjerve, Kristian S; Bjorgaas, Marit R; Lydersen, Stian; and Grill, Valdemar. "Effects of n-3 Fatty Acids In Subjects with Type 2 Diabetes: Reduction of Insulin Sensitivity and Time-Dependent Alteration from Carbohydrate to Fat Oxidation." *American Journal of Clinical Nutrition,* September 2006. 84: 3. 540-550. Online version. Retrieved 11/06/06 from: http://www.ajcn.org/cgi/content/full/84/3/540

Olshansky, Jay S; Passaro, Douglas J; Hershow, Ronald C; Layden, Jennifer; Carnes, Bruce A.; Brody, Jacob; Hayflick, Leonard; Butler, Robert N; Allison, David B; and Ludwig, David S. "Rising Obesity Rates Annihilate Previous Life Span Forecasts." [Electronic version]. *New England Journal of Medicine* 352 (11):1138-1145.(2005, March 17). Retrieved September 19, 2006, from the World Wide Web: http://content.nejm.org/cgi/content/short/352/11/1138

Price, Allen. "Lower Blood Sugar With Bitter Melon: Diabetics in Asia Have Used This Tropical Fruit for Centuries: Herb Brief." *Natural Health,* May-June, 2003; online version. Retrieved 11/05/06 from: http://www.findarticles.com/p/articles/mi_m0NAH/is_4_33/ai_100732342

Przybylski, Roman. "Buckwheat May Be Beneficial For Managing Diabetes." *American Chemical Society.* November 18, 2003. Cited in Medical News Today. Online version. Retrieved 11/04/06 from: http://www.medicalnewstoday.com/medicalnews.php?newsid=4694

Ros, Emilio. "Dietary Cis-Monounsaturated Fatty Acids and Metabolic Control In Type 2 Diabetes." *American Journal of Clinical Nutrition,* September, 2003; 78: 3, 617S-625S, online version. Retrieved 11/03/06 from: http://www.ajcn.org/cgi/reprint/78/3/617S

Ou, Shiyi; Kwok, Kin-chor; Li, Yan; and Fu, Liang. "In Vitro Study of Possible Role of Dietary Fiber in Lowering Postprandial Serum Glucose." 2001; *American Chemical Society,* online abstract. Retrieved 11/04/06 from: http://pubs.acs.org/cgibin/abstract.cgi/jafcau/2001/49/i02/abs/jf000574n.html

Sharma, RD; Sarkar, A; Hazra, DK; Mishra, B; Singh, JB; Sharma, SK; Maheshwari, BB; Maheshwari, PK. Use of "Fenugreek Seed Powder in the Management of Non-insulin Dependent Diabetes Mellitus." *Nutrition Research* (Nutr. Res.). 1996, 16:8, pp. 1331-1339. Cited in Centre National de la Recherche Scientifique. Online version. Retrieved 11/08/06 from: http://cat.inist.fr/?aModele=afficheN&cpsidt=3196194

Trowell, H. "Diabetes Mellitus and Dietary Fiber of Starchy Foods." *American Journal of Clinical Nutrition.* 1978; 31: S53-S57. Online version. Abstract. Retrieved 11/04/06 from: http://www.ajcn.org/cgi/content/abstract/31/10/S53?maxtoshow=&HITS=10&hits=10&RESULTFORMAT=&fulltext=diabetes&searchid=1&FIRSTINDEX=0&sortspec=relevance&resourcetype=HWCIT

Nourishing Your Aging Parents & Yourself

by Edward Bauman, M.Ed., Ph.D.

When I get older, losing my hair
Many years from now
Will you still be sending me a valentine
Birthday greeting, bottle of wine
If I stay out till quarter to three
Will you bar the door
Will you still need me
Will you still feed me
When I'm sixty-four

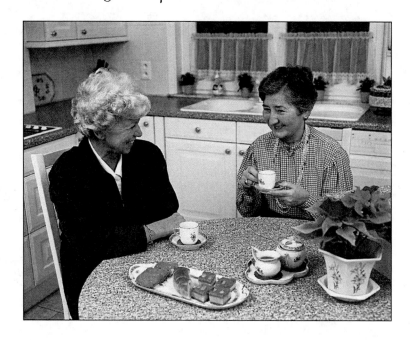

Beetle Paul McCartney was 25 years old when he wrote this song. Today he is 64 and in seemingly excellent health. Each of us is aging, day-by-day, some healthfully, some not so well.

Many baby boomers are finding their own children grown and are taking on the responsibility of caring for mom and dad. Aging parents can require much the same level of care as young children. To help families meet the task nutritionally, I wrote a new verse to the tune of the Beetle song above. Try singing along with me.

Now that you're older
Eating your flax
Keeps you regular
You can have a smoothie nearly every day
With green powder, berries, and whey
Forget the coffee, it's time for tea
You'll be feeling free
Yes, I still need you and I will feed you
When you're eighty-four

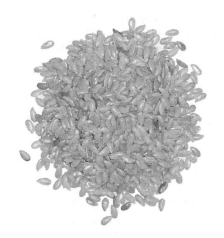

Nourishing Your Aging Parents and Yourself—CONTINUED

What To Do with Aging Parents

As adult children, it's time for us to show up for our parents who nursed us along as infants and did what they could to provide for us. Here are some of the things you can do for your folks:

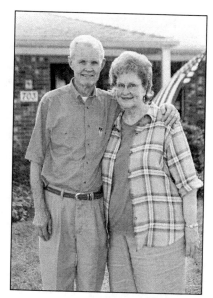

- ▶ Accept the aging process;
- ▶ Identify needs: theirs and yours;
- ▶ Inventory what you have to give;
- ▶ Appreciate the role reversal;
- ▶ Build a support network
- ▶ Mend fences;
- ▶ Honor your commitments; and
- ▶ Make sure they are optimally nourished

Let's use an 84-year-old male parent as an example. Clearly, he is not as sharp as he was in his youth. At this time of life, we might see fading senses, loss of coordination, cognitive decline and signs of dementia, extreme fatigue, depression, increasing resistance and rigidity, diminished social contacts, fear of life and death, and a loss of self esteem. Metabolically, we see diminished appetite, digestion, absorption, muscle mass, bone density, endocrine output, immune capability, and cellular energy production. There may also be excessive complaints, medications to monitor, pain, insomnia, frailty, doctor visits, crisis episodes, financial worries, and irrationality. How can an adult child manage all of this and not be overwhelmed in the process?

Lifestyles for Healthy Aging

If a parent is in his 80s, then the child is likely to be in his or her 50s, give or take a few years. This is the time to jump start a daily, proactive, holistic lifestyle for yourself that includes being:

- ▶ Physically active;
- ▶ Mentally active;
- ▶ Emotionally active;
- ▶ Spiritually active;
- ▶ Socially active; and
- ▶ Nutritionally active.

Health is not a spectator sport. Far too many people expect western medicine to manage their chronic, degenerative health conditions with medication and surgery, but to their dismay, they find it is largely up to them to regain their vitality and well-being. This is true for both the adult child and aging parent. Nutrition is a key to recovery and rejuvenation.

Nourishing Your Aging Parents and Yourself—CONTINUED

Eating For Health™

The *Eating For Health™* model (Bauman, 2006) provides a map of what to eat on a daily basis to provide optimal nutrition. When aging parents become ill, they are often denied the opportunity to eat fresh, local, seasonal, organic foods that are also easy to chew and swallow.

The Bauman College nutrition-based Culinary Arts program trains natural chefs to work with families that include aging parents, preparing appropriate meals in the home or taking them into care facilities, not only to control illnesses such as diabetes or cancer, but to cater to the preferences and pleasure of the clients by preparing the food with love and presenting it with respect and beauty.

All too often, our elders die of malnutrition and a lack of love, rather than heart or kidney failure.

Nutritional Supplements

It is most important for the family to work with a certified clinical nutritionist and medical provider who can properly assess the metabolic and nutritional needs of the aging parent. The research is replete with citations of corrective nutrition to slow the onset and progression of brain and body diseases.

A breakfast smoothie, consisting of whey, flax, green powder, and berries might also include yogurt, coconut, fish oil, l-glutamine, acidophilus, maca, and/or vitamin C. This is far more nourishing than the can of Ensure prescribed by doctors to protect against malnutrition. Other corrective nutrients can diminish pain, suffering, depression, and cognitive decline. These may include digestive enzymes, antioxidants, zinc, magnesium, calcium, chromium, selenium, lipoic acid, and coenzyme Q-10. Of special interest, *GlyceroPhosphoCholine* (GPC) has been used to build cell membranes and mental performance in patients afflicted with stroke or other brain injury.

CONCLUSION

It's high time we shifted away from ignoring and over-medicating our elders, shunting them off to nursing homes with limited care and poor quality food. Our parents are our link with the past and forerunners of how we will be as we age. It's never too late to show up for our parents and advocate for them to receive the best of natural and conventional care. When we commit to nourishing our aging parents, we will likewise notice a profound shift in caring for ourselves and our extended families.

How America's Corn-ucopia
Is Making Us Fat

by Jodi Friedlander, M.S. & Edward Bauman, M.Ed., Ph.D.

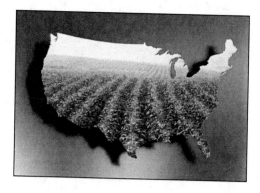

Theories and hypotheses abound as to why the United States is experiencing what many regard as its most serious public health threat, an epidemic of overweight and obesity. Two-thirds of America's adults are overweight or obese and as many as 30 percent of U.S. children are overweight, with childhood obesity more than doubling in the past 25 years. Corresponding with this trend, childhood diabetes has increased ten-fold within the past 20 years (Olshansky et al., 2005). Pollution in our environment, the toxicity of our food supply, our propensity for a couch-potato lifestyle, and super-sized food portions certainly all play a part in the super-sizing of our population. Take a closer look at the contributing causes, though, and one discovers a common denominator underlying all of this: lots of cheap food.

Michael Pollan, food journalist and author of *The Omnivore's Dilemma: A Natural History of Four Meals*, points out that when populations are faced with plentiful and cheap food, they will eat it, and that the average American's daily intake of calories has jumped by more than 10% since 1977 (p. 102). Of all the cheap foods available, Pollan tells us, none is more widespread than corn. He is not referring to sweet summer corn on the cob, nor to corn tortillas or most other foods that are recognizable as corn, but to all of the industrial permutations of corn, such as sweeteners, corn-fed livestock, and an array of processed foods. It is so pervasive in our food supply that if you eat fast foods or packaged foods at all, it is likely that you are eating corn.

Binge Eating of Refined Carbohydrates:
Alcohol and Corn

According to Pollan's research (2002), there have been two periods of epidemic binging in America's history. The first occurred at the turn of the nineteenth century, as a wave of cheap liquor washed over the country and alcohol abuse proliferated, along with its attendant social and health problems. The second era of binging, one that is far more serious, is now upon us, as we eat ourselves literally sick unto death on energy-dense foods lacking in the vital nutrients necessary for health.

What these two eras have in common is an overabundance of corn. Currently comprising about a quarter of our farmland and producing nine billion bushels a year, corn is our single largest crop (Wilson, 2005). This overabundance brings down prices, creating plentiful food at dirt cheap prices. In the early 1800s there were two things you could do with too much corn: feed it to the hogs or distill it into hard liquor (Pollan, 2003). Today we rely on the genius of food technologists to devise "a-maize-ing" ways to fashion our current surplus into various kinds of profitable foodstuffs in ever-larger serving sizes, on which we consumers grow fat.

Political Economy of Corn

Commodity surpluses are common and result from a complex mix of political forces, which in this country include huge subsidy payments to farmers that ultimately encourage overproduction. Corn is our most heavily subsidized crop, to the tune of $10 billion a year (Wilson, 2005). There is a unique component to the corn subsidy story. The European Union and a growing number of other countries have refused to purchase *genetically modified* (GMO)

How America's Corn-ucopia Is Making Us Fat—CONTINUED

foods. It is estimated that between 3% and 5% of our sweet corn crop is GMO, and since it goes into the mix with non-GMO corn, these countries steadfastly refuse to purchase our corn.

Jeffrey Smith, in his best-selling book *Seeds of Deception*, reported that by 2003 U.S. corn exports (including feed corn) to the European Union were down 99.4% (p. 153). This means we've got a lot of extra corn on our hands and our huge industrial-farming corporations are desperately trying to get it sold and into the food supply. The big profits, though, are made not by selling the corn but by creating value-added processed foods.

High Fructose Corn Sweetener and Obesity: No Accident

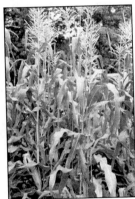

Enter modern science. It is well-known that *high-fructose corn syrup* (HFCS), an inexpensive, highly concentrated product synthesized from cornstarch, is widely used in the food industry, most notably as the primary sweetener in soft drinks and baked goods. What is less well known is that its usage increased 1000% between 1970, when it entered our food supply, and 1990 (Bray et al., 2004). This vast increase in usage far surpasses that of any other food or food group and is largely due to its incredibly low price. In their insatiable hunger for higher profits, food manufacturers add increasing amounts of it to their products in ever-increasing portion sizes. Instead of the once common eight-ounce soft drink, we are now more likely to find a 20-ounce (or bigger) size.

HFCS currently represents 40% of sweeteners added to foods and beverages, and it is conservatively estimated that the average rate of consumption is 132 daily calories for everyone over the age of two (Bray et al., 2004). For heavy consumers, this figure increases to more than 300 calories per day. This works out to an average range of about 10-20% of daily calories from HFCS.

The skyrocketing of HFCS in the food supply has paralleled our nation's rapid increase in obesity. Here's why. Bray et al.'s 2004 study, published in the *American Journal of Clinical Nutrition*, reported that HFCS, and fructose in general, metabolizes differently than glucose and sucrose. This study revealed that fructose does not elicit a response from insulin, does not increase leptin production, and does not suppress ghrelin production. In short, it short-circuits the hormonal process that signals satiation and helps regulate food intake and body weight. Instead, fructose is sent directly to the liver, bypassing the intermediary breakdown steps that occur with sucrose. The liver's response to the fructose is to generate new fat cells, which it then dumps into the bloodstream as triglycerides.

Another study, coming to the same conclusion, found that a diet high in fructose elevates triglyceride levels shortly after eating far more significantly than a diet high in sucrose, particularly in men (Critser, 2004, p. 137). Muscles, bombarded by triglycerides, will develop insulin resistance rather quickly. A study done on golden hamsters, which metabolize fats very much like humans do, found that insulin resistance developed just a few weeks after starting a high-fructose diet (Critser, 2004, p. 137). Overall, such studies have found that high fructose intake changes the way we metabolize fats, causing us to store fat and burn sugar.

Glut on the Market of Calorie-Rich/Nutrient-Poor Processed Foods

Adding to the obesity problem, people who drink HFCS-sweetened drinks tend to take in too many calories overall (evidently believing that calories don't count when you're not chewing). Fructose is also the main sugar found in fruit juices, which, while naturally occurring, does not have the accompanying fruit fiber to slow its uptake. Add

How America's Corn-ucopia Is Making Us Fat—CONTINUED

this to our off-the-charts HFCS consumption and the primary role of fructose in the obesity epidemic becomes obvious.

Where does the rest of the corn go? By visiting the Corn Refiners Association website – **www.corn.org** – one learns that there are many other sweeteners made from corn, including maltose, maltodextrin, dextrose, glucose, and crystalline fructose. Who could fault even the most intrepid label-reading consumer for not knowing this? The list of corn-derived products also includes amino acids, vitamins, monosodium glutamate, mono- and di-glycerides, citric and lactic acids, cornstarch and other starches, as well as vegetable oils, margarines, and shortenings. Thousands of supermarket staples contain products made from corn, mostly in the form of starches.

Corn, along with soy, is ubiquitous in the marketplace. Though our processed foods have the semblance of diversity, corn and soy permeate them all. When not organically produced, both crops require large quantities of pesticides and herbicides to thrive. If toxins in the food supply also contribute to weight gain, as many scientists believe, then these two dominant crops are certainly suspect.

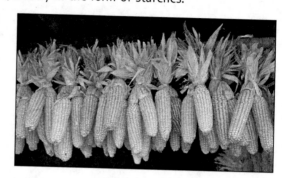

Undiagnosed Corn Allergies

Corn may cause allergic symptoms as a contactant (talcs, bath oils and powders, starched clothing, and corn adhesives); as an inhalant (fumes from vegetable forms of corn as they cook); and as an ingestant (corn and corn products that are eaten). Corn-sensitive people are advised to avoid all forms of corn for a minimum of 30 days, and then to reintroduce whole corn products (corn on the cob, then organic tortillas) and watch for reactions, such as fatigue, irritability, inflammation, etc. (Krohn, 2000; pp. 108-112).

Always read labels! When inquiring about whether a product contains corn, ask about corn flour, oil, starch, and sugar (dextrose), as well as HFCS. Vegetable oils need not be identified on commercial labels, so sensitive people should assume that commercial products containing vegetable oil may contain processed corn oil. Likewise, sugars do not have to be labeled as derived from corn, cane, or beet. To be safe, then, it is wise to avoid all commercially sweetened products.

GMO Corn-Fed Animals and Fatty Acids

But there's more. We feed a lot of corn (and soy)—much of both genetically modified—to cattle, including those we eat and those whose milk we consume. While little is known about how this affects dairy products, studies have shown that the fat content of our meat differs radically from that of cattle fed entirely on pasturage. Grass-fed beef is significantly lower in overall fat content, lower in saturated fat content, and higher in polyunsaturated fat content (Daley et al., 2006a). A joint study by California State University, Chico and the University of California Cooperative Extension Service found that beef from cattle fed solely on grass provided a healthier ratio of Omega-6 to Omega-3 fats—3:1 versus about 20:1 in grain-fed beef.

Professor Tony Hulbert, PhD., a professor of biology at the University of Wollongong in Australia, has been performing experiments with fatty acids on cell membranes. He has found that the Omega-3 fats, because they make cell membranes runnier, allow molecules to pass in and out more quickly (Blanch, 2005). This finding strongly sug-

How America's Corn-ucopia Is Making Us Fat—CONTINUED

gests that the sped up transit time translates to an increased metabolic rate. He has, in fact, found that wild animals that eat Omega-3 rich diets have very high metabolisms. Since our hunter-gatherer days, when it is estimated that our Omega-6 to Omega-3 ratio was 1:1, the human diet has moved away from Omega-3 fatty acids and now favors Omega-6 fats, as well as damaged fats that our bodies were never designed to ingest.

The Chico/UC study's grass-fed cattle also contained up to 50% more conjugated linoleic acid (CLA) than the grain-fed cattle (Daley et al., 2006b). Another study has shown that CLA, in amounts above 3.4 grams per day, reduces adipose tissue stores and reduces Body Fat Mass in human study subjects (Blankson et al., 2000). This combination of lowered metabolic rate and lowered intake of CLA when consuming grain-fed beef may be a big piece of the weight gain puzzle. And remember, these cattle are not fed grain because it's a healthful part of their diets (grain is actually too high in protein for ruminants and makes them ill [Pearce, J., ruminant specialist; private communication, August 26, 2006]) but because it makes them gain weight, and quickly. For us humans, this form of corn has been refined and processed inside a cow rather than in a manufacturing plant, but once again we're consuming a highly refined corn product.

The same holds true for commercial chickens, even those produced organically, except that chickens don't become sick from this diet. Corn and soy are now also being fed to our farm-raised fish and for the very same reason: it makes them grow big and fat very quickly on cheap feed. It also skews their fat ratios, completely negating the reason we've all started eating cold-water fish in the first place — for their Omega-3 fatty acids. Buyer beware.

Corny is no Longer Funny

Overall, it's a corny country we inhabit. Our "amber waves of grain," once known as the fat of the land, now contribute greatly to the land of the fat. Our large food manufacturers and meat producers, under the guise of producing appealing and diverse foods, are in reality merely processing and refining products made from corn and other energy-dense commodity foods.

To change this situation would mean the undoing of governmental laws regulating food subsidies and the political favoring of large corporations. It is on an individual level that consumers exercise the most power. As nutrition professionals, it is incumbent upon us to teach our clients to be more conscious of where our foods come from so that they, too, can consciously make wise choices for both physical and political reasons.

By adopting and promoting a whole-foods, predominantly organic diet, we never have to worry about overly refined commodity foods making us fat, or about the toxins so pervasive within them. We will be eating a far more diversified and healthful diet, and we will be making a powerful political statement with our food choices. According to Michael Pollan (Wagenvoord, 2004), there already has been some reform in the food supply due to consumer demand. He contends that the food industry is very sensitive to this demand, as demonstrated by how many of the large companies now have an organic division and by how much more capital than ever before is going into organic agriculture. He says:

"If consumers make good choices, the industry will respond."

Let's hope he's right.

How America's Corn-ucopia Is Making Us Fat—CONTINUED

REFERENCES

Anonymous (2002). "A brief history of the corn refining industry." *Corn Refiners Association.* Retrieved September 17, 2006 from the World Wide Web: www.corn.org/web/history.htm.

Anonymous (2002). "Products made from corn." *Corn Refiners Association.* Retrieved September 17, 2006 from the World Wide Web: www.corn.org/web/products.htm.

Blanch, D. (2005, March 28). "Eat fat to get thin." *ABC Radio Australia.* Retrieved September 18, 2006 from the World Wide Web: www.abc.net.au/ra/innovations/stories/s1334086.htm.

Blankson, H., Stakkestad, J.A., Fagertun, H., Thom, E., Wadstein, J., and Gudmundsen, O. (2000). "Conjugated linoleic acid reduces body fat mass in overweight and obese humans." [Electronic version]. *Journal of Nutrition*, 130: 2943-2948. Retrieved September 17, 2006 from the World Wide Web: jn.nutrition.org/cgi/content/full/130/12/2943.

Bray, George A.; Neilsen, Samara Joy; and Popkin, Barry M. "Consumption of high-fructose corn syrup in beverages may play a role in the epidemic of obesity." [Electronic version]. *American Journal of Clinical Nutrition* 79 (4): 537. Retrieved September 16, 2006,= from the World Wide Web: www.ajcn.org/cgi/content/full/79/4/537.

Critser, G. (2004). "What the extra calories do to you." *Fat land.* (pp. 136-140). New York: Houghton Mifflin.

Daley, C.A., A.Abbott, P. Doyle, G. Nader, and S. Larson. California State University, College of Agriculture, University of California Cooperative Extension Service. (2006, May). "Effect of ration on lipid profiles in beef." [Electronic version]. Retrieved September 16, 2006 from the World Wide Web: www.csuchico.edu/agr/grassfedbeef/health-benefits/index.html.

Daley, C.A., A.Abbott, P. Doyle, G. Nader, and S. Larson. California State University, College of Agriculture, University of California Cooperative Extension Service. (2006, May). A literature review of the value-added nutrients found in grass-fed beef products. [Electronic version]. Retrieved September 16, 2006, from the World Wide Web: www.csuchico.edu/agr/grass-fedbeef/health-benefits/index.html.

Krohn, J. (2000). *Allergy Relief and Prevention.* Hartley and Marx Publishers. Vancouver, BC.

Olshansky, S. Jay et al. (2005, March 17). "Rising obesity rates annihilate previous life span forecasts." [Electronic version]. *New England Journal of Medicine* 352 (11):1138-1145. Retrieved September 19, 2006 from the World Wide Web: www.merco-la.com/2005/apr/2/obesity_rates.htm.

Pollan, M. (2002, July 19). "When a crop becomes king." [Electronic version]. *New York Times Magazine.* Retrieved September 15, 2006, from the World Wide Web: http://query.nytimes.com/gst/fullpage.html?sec=health&tres=9C05E5DE113 F93AA2579C05E5DE1139F93AA25754C0A9649C8B63.

Pollan, M. (2003, October 12). "The way we live now: the (agri)cultural contradictions of obesity." [Electronic version]. *New York Times Magazine.* Retrieved September 15, 2006 from the World Wide Web: http://query.nytimes.com/gst/fullpage.html?sec=health&tres=9A0DE2D61E3CF931A25753C1A9659C8B63.

Pollan, M. (2006). "Industrial corn." In *The Omnivore's Dilemma: A Natural History of Four Meals.* (pp. 15-119). New York: Penguin Press.

Smith, Jeffrey M. (2003). "Government by the industry, for the industry." In *Seeds of Deception.* (p. 153). Fairfield, Iowa: Yes!

Wagenvoord, H. (2004, September/October). Interview: Michael Pollan. "The cheapest calories make you the fattest, a "food-chain journalist" looks for stories in our meals." *Sierra Magazine* online. Retrieved September 16, 2006 from the World Wide Web: www.sierraclub.org/sierra/200409/interview.asp.

Wilson, K. (2005, July 20) "The tragic abuse of corn." *Organic Consumers Association.* Retrieved September 18, 2006 from the World Wide Web: www.organicconsumers.org/Corn/abused072705.cfm

BIOGRAPHIES

A once-and-future student of Ed Bauman, M.Ed., PhD., Jodi Friedlander, M.S., earned her Master's degree in Holistic Nutrition from Clayton College of Natural Health. She lives in Tehachapi, California with her husband, Scott, and their dog and three cats. She maintains a private nutrition consulting practice, specializing in issues of weight gain, hormone imbalance, and stress disorders. She also writes a monthly nutrition newspaper column, lectures, and teaches private nutrition classes. She keeps her life in balance with gardening, hiking, biking, running, rock climbing, and yoga. She is constantly asked, "Where the heck is Tehachapi?" She can be contacted at: **jfriedlander05@yahoo.com**

Edward Bauman, M.Ed., Ph.D. is the director of Bauman College: Holistic Nutrition and Culinary Arts, which has three classroom campuses in Northern California and an innovative distance learning program. Ed is committed to bringing the message of *Eating For Health*™ to a wider audience to reverse the tendencies toward mindless over-consumption of sickening foods. He can be reached at: **edb@baumancollege.org**

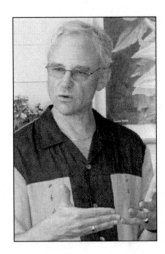

Healthy Weight Loss & Good Nutrition:
An Interview with Dr. Ed Bauman

By Dennis Hughes, Share Guide Publisher

Edward Bauman, M.Ed., Ph.D. has been a ground-breaking leader in the field of whole foods nutrition, holistic health, and community health promotion. He is the Founder and Director of Bauman College for Holistic Nutrition and Culinary Arts, based in Penngrove, California. His approach is non-judgmental and collaborative, allowing people to make their own choices based on individual needs and preferences.

D.H. Dr. Bauman, there are many different programs now for weight loss, and it gets confusing. Some say that you should drastically reduce your carb intake, and some say it's fat that's the problem and carbs are okay. How do we know what's true?

E.B. Just restricting fats or carbohydrates will not work. People need to clear out the chemicals, add the nutrients, and develop an internal practice that enables them to feel happy and peaceful. There's a simple equation to use: too many calories, plus too many chemicals, minus nutrients, minus internal peace and balance, equals poor metabolism and weight gain. In regards to too many calories, you can have too many calories from protein, or too many calories from fat, or too many calories from soft drinks. Excess calories can come from any source. The addition of artificial colors, fats, preservatives, additives, and industrial waste into the food supply has gotten into people's tissues and has disrupted metabolism and contributed to enormous fat gain. This can happen even on a limited-calorie diet. Animal products tend to concentrate fat-soluble compounds in the environment, so limiting fat on the one hand would limit the amount of foreign chemicals, but healthy fats are essential for hormonal balance and nerve balance.

The other part of the equation is the nutritional deficiencies that are numerous in a standard American diet. This doesn't even have to be a bad diet. If you're eating take-out food, or food that is not natural, wholesome, organic, and seasonal, it's going to be limited in nutrients. The recent *National Health and Nutrition Evaluation Survey* showed that 97% of people in the United States were deficient in the essential fatty acids. These are found largely in fish, in flax and other seeds like chia or hemp, and in algae. The survey also showed that 60% were deficient in magnesium.

Another variable is stress, which is very disruptive to the digestive system, the nervous system, the hormonal system, and the fat-burning system. When people are stressed, they store calories. So even with proper exercise, a good diet, and clean living, if people are unable to find a level of peace, their brains and nervous systems are constantly in fear, which tends to trigger weight gain.

So again, it's very complex why people are overweight.

Healthy Weight Loss & Good Nutrition:
An Interview with Dr. Ed Bauman—CONTINUED

D.H. Some people, like Barry Sears with his Zone Diet, say that the important point is how you balance carbs, proteins, and fat at each meal.

E.B. People are different, so I think the possibilities are more varied than the approach of the *Zone Diet*. Looking at nutrient density is helpful, which would lean more towards the Zone system, meaning that having a strong mixture of fats and proteins relative to carbohydrates within a meal, a person would have a higher satiation, which means they'd be satisfied. People could eat a smaller amount of food and have it sustain them longer without them getting hungry.

I think that within the higher protein models, calorie restriction is a vital component, which some people realize, some people don't. This also explains why there was some success with the higher protein diets such as the Atkins diet. People were saturating themselves with fats and proteins, balancing that out with vegetables, and minimizing the intake of fruits and grains and other carbohydrates. But for that to be successful, they had to work within a caloric structure of 1200–1600 calories. If people ate that same balance of nutrients but consumed 2000 calories (which is the normal recommendation for an average-size man), they wouldn't lose weight.

One part of the problem is the difference between men and women — the standards don't necessarily look at women being smaller and having less muscle mass versus men. There also needs to be some consciousness about caloric intake, because a lot of people are somewhat ignorant of how many calories they're getting from their foods. They're getting bigger portions of foods, and they're eating in a stressed out way.

D.H. Some nutritionists say the easiest way to lose weight is to eat several small meals throughout the day, rather than three big ones. But others, such as Jack LaLanne, say that you should never snack between meals. What's your opinion?

E.B. It's still going to boil down to caloric intake, nutrient intake, and whether or not people are metabolizing well. Certainly the element of exercise and physical activity has got to be part of the weight-loss program. There is no weight loss without physical energy expenditure. But people who eat poorly are not going to lose weight, even with tons of exercise, because they're going to be missing certain nutrients. They'll plateau, which is what normally happens. For people who drop their calories and push up their exercise, at some point they'll get a thermogenic effect, and they'll be pretty excited. Then if their nutrients are limited they'll plateau, and then they'll start to put weight back on. They'll exercise more, they'll still plateau, then they'll panic. That's where nutritional guidance is very important, to look for what's missing. Is it the fatty acids, or zinc, magnesium, B vitamins, amino acids — or something peculiar to that person on a genetic basis? I don't generalize for every person. There's no single formula that works for everyone. People are biochemically individual. There are also psycho-social variables.

Healthy Weight Loss & Good Nutrition:
An Interview with Dr. Ed Bauman—CONTINUED

D.H. Some weight loss experts say that you should never eat late in the evening, and others say that late-night snacks are fine.

E.B. It depends on how late people stay up in terms of whether or not it's optimal for them to have an evening snack, and then it depends on what the snack is. If you have dinner at six, and you go to bed at ten, you're probably okay. But if you have dinner at six and you go to bed at midnight, that's a long stretch. So if somebody gets beyond four hours without eating and they need some fuel, then having a snack would make sense... but not ice cream and chocolate chip cookies! A good snack might be yogurt and fruit, or some popcorn with nutritional yeast, or a little toast with almond butter. But again, it would be just enough to stabilize the blood sugar, not a large amount.

D.H. Some say you can eat whatever you want, as long as you exercise rigorously everyday.

E.B. Well, there are people who are very oriented towards physical activity. Their main mode of expression is through physical activity, so they're the ones who will exercise several hours a day, or whose work is physically demanding. But they are not the majority. Extreme exercise is not important for everyone, or even beneficial for everyone. However, getting no exercise is detrimental to everyone. So what we have to deal with here is exercise resistance. As people get older and have injuries and illnesses, their exercise tolerance goes down, which means they really have difficulty sustaining exercise for more than a short time, such as 10, 15, or 20 minutes. But the benefit of exercise is actually greater for someone with low exercise tolerance. If someone who's really out of shape goes for a 10-minute walk, they get more benefit than somebody who's highly in shape who does a 45-minute bike ride. So the general population needs to be coached and nurtured and encouraged to build up exercise tolerance, just like people need to be coached and nurtured to make better food choices. It usually takes six months for people to internalize this and make changes, even when they say, "Yes, I'm ready to get well!"

A holistic viewpoint looks at things as an entire system across an entire lifetime. Unfortunately, most people who are writing books are saying, "Better Weight in 30 Days." People are not looking at this as a lifetime practice; they're looking at it as a short-term commitment. That's not the approach that I present to people. When you talk about this method versus that method, it is still somebody else's external program that you're trying to adopt, and at some point it will fail to have relevance for you.

D.H. Some nutritionists say that sugar is the real problem, and you should completely eliminate it, including sweet vegetables like carrots and beets.

E.B. You get people who are into black-and-white thinking, but that's not my view. The idea is to look for balance and proportion in nutrient density. It's not the individual ingredient that's the issue. Carrots are a good food, yams are a good food, even cane sugar has B vitamins and chromium in it if it's not refined. But if one is eating out of a box, there's likely to be too much added sugar or artificial sweetener. People are very seduced by the sweet taste. They expect sweet and salt, and a certain amount of fat for mouth feel, so the whole food industry is pandering to that and it's a problem.

Healthy Weight Loss & Good Nutrition:
An Interview with Dr. Ed Bauman—CONTINUED

However, you can take things to an extreme. What if you buy a yogurt and it has organic milk and it has organic fruit, but it has cane sugar as the third ingredient? There are people who'd say to get rid of that item because it has sugar. But the fruit has sugar in it, and even the yogurt has sugar in it. Inevitably, people are going to have exposure to sugar, whether it's natural or artificial. What I'm saying is don't eat food that has sugar as the first ingredient, and don't have your meal be predominant in high-glycemic foods. You can eat yams, and carrots, and beets as long as you eat them with a lean protein and a good fat such as olive oil, avocado, or almonds.

D.H. Regarding sugar, aren't stevia and xylitol healthier alternatives?

E.B. Well, they're natural. They will burn up in the system, and they don't create an adverse effect, but they could be over-consumed, as well, because of the sweetness that they bring. I would prefer that people actually use whole foods rather than food extracts or concentrates. Stevia is condensed from 100 pounds of stevia leaves into one ounce of stevia liquid or concentrate. You're not getting the whole plant so you're not getting the other phytonutrients. I would prefer that you had a drop of honey or maple syrup in your tea, rather than use stevia.

Because of calorie phobia and the phobia of sugar, people end up with a packaged alternative to what you could get in a natural way. I'm not saying stevia or xylitol are harmful, but they're expensive and they're energy-demanding — having to make it from leaves to powder to package. You're adding steps in the ecological process that are somewhat unnecessary. The real problem is not sugar; it's the over-consumption of sugar and the over-refinement of sugar.

D.H. Many books say "This is the easiest, most innovative diet plan," even if it's the same recycled knowledge.

E.B. Unfortunately, people are turning everything into a commodity. They're either selling a book, or selling a product, or selling a program, and they're not really teaching principles of health and nutrition to people. Then people get into this mentality of "I'm cheating now, I'm not following the program." That creates a certain level of guilt. I don't approach it that way. I'm teaching people about natural foods and a natural lifestyle, with some room for people to experiment within healthy choices.

I have a system called the **Four Levels of Eating,** which I think is very helpful for people. The first level is *Eating for Pleasure,* and you're basically eating to make yourself happy and to minimize pain. The second level is *Eating for Energy.* At this level, you're just eating to stay full, but it's more than just pleasure and pain. You have to take care of your blood sugar, but you're eating on the run. But after a couple of decades of eating just for pleasure and energy, people get sick. They look in the mirror; they don't look well and they don't feel well. That puts them into the third level, *Eating for Recovery.* This level is a diet program. It might be high-fat, low-fat, high-carb, blood type — there's discrimination involved. There are dos and don'ts, but they're somebody else's idea. Usually after three months, people plateau on these pro-

Healthy Weight Loss & Good Nutrition:
An Interview with Dr. Ed Bauman—CONTINUED

grams – they get sick of it. People shop around and they follow program A, and program B, and program C, and then after awhile they think "this is crazy," because they haven't gained their own sense of understanding. Then they usually just go back to random eating.

The fourth level is what I call *Eating For Health.* This is where you begin to look at your patterns and at what type of foods and what kind of lifestyle really works for you. You're making choices among good things, rather than between a good ingredient and a bad ingredient. You're eating with some discrimination, moderation, and consciousness, and you have purpose in what you're doing. You realize that you're taking care of your body for the long haul. So if somebody says "Want some ice cream and cake?", you say "No thanks" – but not because you're on a rigid diet or you're not eating fats or carbs. It's because at that moment, you realize it's not a particularly high choice. Or you might have a little bit and then say "that's enough." The mentality is different. You're caring for yourself, and you're looking at where your own limits are and what your own needs are.

Typically at this level you're working with an advisor. They'll say these are the nutrients, or the foods, or the herbs that will help you with your issues around thyroid, around insulin, around blood sugar, or around muscle building, etc. But there's no "cheating." The locus of control is within yourself. If you overeat, or you make a bad choice, you take that into consideration and you don't repeat it. This shift in thinking opens you up to a wide panorama of healthy choices, rather than a limited "diet." It's working towards maturity and self-actualization, rather than looking at dependency and being told what to do by yet another expert.

Mastery is what life is about, and nutrition is one of the paths that takes people into understanding themselves and being self-actualized. Then you are able to share and impart knowledge with other people without telling them what to do – because what works for you is not necessarily what's going to work for them.

D.H. Are there really supplements that are effective in helping people burn fat and lose weight, or do you think they're all a fraud?

E.B. If you exercise and take supplements, the supplements will help you lose weight. But if you don't have a good diet and a good lifestyle, then even if you take good supplements you probably won't lose weight. I've worked with hundreds of people who have bought everything there is under the sun, but they really didn't have the inner life worked out at all. If they began to shift their food choices, then the chromium, or the CLA, or whatever they were taking could help.

In essence, the supplements prime the pump. They might stimulate a metabolic effect, or they might help control your appetite. But at a certain point, you'll basically reach tolerance with those substances; your body will no longer respond to those cues. I'm not against people taking supplements, particularly nutrients that will help improve their metabolism, but they have to do it within a holistic approach to diet and lifestyle if they're going to expect any kind of return on their investment.

Healthy Weight Loss & Good Nutrition:
An Interview with Dr. Ed Bauman—CONTINUED

D.H. You are a big proponent of fasting. How often and for how long do you recommend fasting?

E.B. When you say the word "fasting," most people think it means consuming only water, but I am not an advocate of water fasting. For 20 years I've led people on supervised juice fasts that involve organic fruit and vegetable juices, herbal teas, and mineral broths, which are soup mixes without the vegetables, just the broth. It's really a modified cleansing, rejuvenating program, rather than a pure fast. I recommend people do a major fast one week a year, during the warm weather time. For an entire week, get off of solid food. Then once each season, do it again for a 3- to 5-day period. For someone who wants to continue to carry it forward, do it one day a week. That's for someone who's really highly motivated or who has a particular health need to do so. But seasonal influences and health issues are very important, so it depends on the individual.

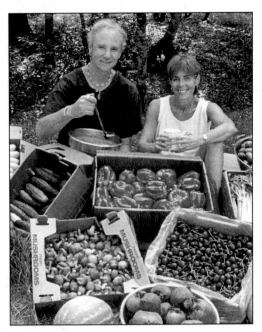

Retreating Into Health: Vitality Fasting™ for Healing & Detoxification

by Edward Bauman, M.Ed., Ph.D.

I have had the pleasure of leading *Vitality Fasting Retreats*™ for the past twenty years. In that time, I have fasted each spring and summer with groups ranging in size from 15 to 48 participants. These residential retreats are held in a beautiful natural setting, away from the noise, food, stress and responsibilities of everyday life.

The program provides a full day and evening schedule of health-promoting activities. The mornings flow from yoga to meditation, group juice preparation, a sharing circle and guided exercise. Afternoons include hiking, swimming, hot tubbing, arts, crafts and optional private nutrition consultations and massage. A variety of health and nutrition classes are offered in the evenings.

Abstaining from solid foods, being in nature, living in community with kindred souls and having ample time and space for private reflection nurtures a deep rejuvenating process at every level of one's being.

What is a Fast?

Clinically speaking, fasting is abstinence from solid food. The most absolute fast is to subsist on air alone. Next on the simplicity scale is consuming only distilled or purified water. Then, there are several varieties of juice fasts, such as the "Master Cleanser," first introduced by Stanley Burroughs, N.D., which prescribes a daily beverage of fresh lemon and water mixed with a measured amount of maple syrup and cayenne pepper.

Over the years, I have perfected the *Vitality Fast*™, which utilizes nutrient-dense liquids, including:

▶ Fresh, seasonal, organic juices;
▶ Warm mineral broths containing sea vegetables, flax seeds and savory culinary spices; and
▶ Herbal teas that address seasonal, group and individual needs.

Consuming a variety of liquid foods provides the body with essential nutrients to both cleanse and rejuvenate tissues and organs.

Recently, I have expanded my fasting program with specially formulated products that protect against pathological detoxification in people for whom liquid fasting is too stressful.

I have also developed a potent phytonutrient powder called *Vital Scoop*™ for fasters to mix in water, tea, broth or juice. It contains whey from grass fed cows, a blend of green foods that include spirulina, chlorella, wheat grass, barley grass, sea vegetables and flora, plus flax seeds and carefully selected organic fruit and seed extracts. Taken as directed, *Vital Scoop*™ supports blood sugar, organ, endocrine and nerve function to aide tissue cleansing. It also provides a level of cellular nutrition that promotes a fresh, natural vitality.

Retreating Into Health: Vitality Fasting™ for Healing & Detoxification—CONTINUED

Maintaining cellular nutrient balance while fasting mitigates detoxification symptoms and re-calibrates one's mental, emotional and spiritual energetics. Fasters come away from retreats feeling that they resonate at a stronger and more pure frequency. Being immersed in nature and supported with superfood beverages, positive leadership and dynamic health practices leads to a remarkable sense of wellness.

Fasters come to understand that this way of being — not the chaotic, toxic, stressful money-mad culture we left behind — is "real life."

Internal and External Cleansing

Vitality Fasting™ supports deep cleansing of the organs of elimination — the liver, bowel, lymph, skin, lungs, and kidneys. There are several components of this process, in addition to the consumption of deeply nourishing beverages. I instruct participants on the benefits and mechanics of self-administered enemas to expedite the release of solid waste. Using a dry brush for massage and a tongue scraper to clear bacterial waste in the mouth further enable the body to slough off layers of dead cells, allowing fresh and vibrant cells to replace them. Getting adequate exercise and rest are other keys to the success of *Vitality Fasting*™.

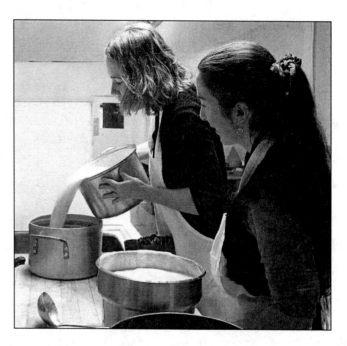

Maintaining Balance

One of the challenges of the fasting process is to remain centered, grounded, and present to the moment. When one takes in less food, blood sugar becomes less stable until the body shifts into an adaptive fasting metabolism. Until one adjusts metabolically and can manage the stress of eating less and detoxifying more, light-headedness, fatigue, and irritability are likely to be experienced.

Often, first-time fasters can't easily let go of their conditioned attachments to work, family, politics, television and other material matters. A fast is best accomplished in a natural retreat setting that allows one to connect more deeply with nature, spirit, peace and quiet.

Detoxification

During the course of our normal lives, the body is in a constant state of ingestion, digestion, assimilation and elimination. *Vitality Fasting*™ minimizes the intake and digestion of food, giving the digestive system a rest. The soothing, healing, alkaline-forming minerals and phytonutrients provided by the freshly made teas, juices and broths free the intestinal mucosa of both food and chemical antigens — substances that provoke an immune response, causing inflammation and tissue degradation.

Retreating Into Health: Vitality Fasting™ for Healing & Detoxification—CONTINUED

Pure, fresh, liquid food requires few enzymes to digest and provides significant amounts of enzyme precursors, such as potassium, magnesium, zinc, Vitamin C and the B-complex vitamins. Juices replenish depleted reserves of nutrients in the liver, pancreas and gut — nutrients needed for optimal digestion, assimilation and blood sugar regulation. A fast is a terrific digestive tune-up for a sluggish system.

As blood is recharged with mineral-rich nutrients, it delivers them to body systems that have been chronically acidic and suffering from free radical damage, or oxidative stress. Once pH balance is restored, cells and tissues slough off metabolic waste and cell debris. This can include stored lipid-soluble environmental toxins, carcinogens and heavy metals such as mercury, lead, arsenic and cadmium.

A well-fortified fasting immune system will target areas of chronic infection and, with the support of therapeutic herbs, diminish the variety and toxicity of pathogenic organisms and their waste products.

Vitality Fasting™ accelerates the assimilation of nutrients and the elimination of waste. The combined effect of skin brushing, guided energetic exercises such as yoga and Tai Chi, hydro-therapy, massage and self-administered enemas is a gentle and thorough cleansing of the entire body with few unpleasant side effects.

Typically, a faster will experience an initial cleansing cycle within three days and feel suddenly light, clear and energized. As the body continues to slough off impurities, less sanguine feelings may surface, only to give way to another cycle of clearing and lightness, typically at days 5, 7, and 10.

Supervision and Breaking the Fast

An experienced fasting supervisor can help fasters navigate any changes in body, mind and emotion they experience, and can guide them in deciding when it is time to break the fast and resume eating solid foods. Fasters often don't want to come "down" and return to the world they call home, which now seems unreal. There is justifiable concern about falling back into the traps of living in a hectic, polluted and confusing world.

Fortunately, the crucial support of friendships formed and lessons learned during *Vitality Fasting*™ are deep and enduring. Fasting is a time-honored holistic practice that allows one to regularly step out of stress and toxicity. It promotes the practice of living well within, manifesting peace for oneself and others.

I advise people who are not fasting to liquefy their solid foods by eating slowly, chewing well, and blessing their food, friends, families, and Mother Nature with every bite.

Namasté!

Ed Bauman, M.Ed., Ph.D. is the director for Bauman College: Holistic Nutrition and Culinary Arts; Bauman Nutrition clinic (www.BaumanNutrition.com) in Penngrove, California; and seasonal *Vitality Fasting Retreats.* His fasting mentors include Drs. Paavo Airola, Henry Biehler, Bernard Jensen, and Ann Wigmore and comedian turned natural health advocate Dick Gregory. Ed is a much-loved nutrition and health instructor, fasting leader and community health advocate. He was a three-term president of NANP and is now focusing on integrating holistic nutrition professionals into schools, communities and the clinical health delivery system. For fun, Ed enjoys music, sports, spiritual practice and pondering his next lifetime of pure play in an enlightened world.

PART TWO:
Therapeutic Foods

Along about 400 BC, Hippocrates, the father of modern medicine, stated:

> *"Leave thy drugs in the chemist's pot
> and let food be thy medicine."*

Today, nearly 2500 years later, this message needs to appear frequently on television to offset the shameful advertising practices of the pharmaceutical, beer, and fast food companies.

Foods, not drugs, provide the body with the nutrients it needs to recover from illness and injury. The fresher the food, the better it will be for our health. The richer the soil and water from which the food came, the more therapeutic benefit the food will provide.

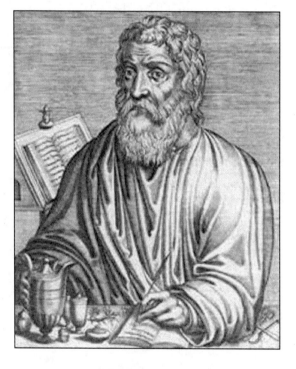

Everything is as healthy as what it ate and absorbed. A healthy chicken will lay healthy eggs. A chicken cooped up and not allowed to eat healthy scratch and feed will not provide the nutritional value we expect based on charts and marketing literature. Look to the natural colors, flavors, and aromas of fresh foods as indicators of their therapeutic value.

In 2006, the *Journal of the American Medical Association* (JAMA) reported that more than 120,000 deaths per year in the United States were due to improper medical treatment. That makes medical care the third leading cause of death for Americans. Natural healing, on the other hand, does not put us at the mercy of conventional treatments like drugs and surgery. Rather, it is based on the principle that all sentient beings depend on the same things in order to live well: sunshine, fresh air, pure water, fresh and uncontaminated foods, physical activity, rest, touch, and love.

Introduction—CONTINUED

The vast majority of people I have met who are seeking nutritional advice to overcome health challenges grew up eating enriched, sweetened cereals soaked with milk from cows who were given growth hormones and antibiotics. They drank soda that contained 12 teaspoons of refined sugar per 12-ounce can; ate candy, chips, cookies, and crackers daily; and were not offered a wide selection of fresh, organic vegetables and fruits. As a result, they became overfed and undernourished. The result is today's epidemic of obesity, diabetes, cardiovascular disease, and cancer. How can drugs or surgery effectively reverse these conditions?

Therapeutic foods — such as avocados, blueberries, flax, broccoli, and wild salmon — are rich in unprocessed proteins, healthy fats, and complex carbohydrates. They also provide a wide range of antioxidants and phytonutrients that protect the body from environmental toxins and metabolic waste. All natural, organic foods can be therapeutic if they are eaten at the peak of freshness and are properly prepared.

In this section, I present a number of therapeutic foods to serve as examples of how a healthy diet can promote growth and healing. I also discuss a variety of spices — such as ginger, oregano, and rosemary — that contain important health-promoting factors. Consuming these foods on a regular basis can help prevent or reverse the diseases that plague us.

Heavyweight Healing Foods

AVOCADO

Although the creamy rich Haas avocados are generally available throughout the year, they are the most abundant and at their best during the spring and summer in California and in October in Florida. During the fall and winter months you can find Fuerto, Zutano and Bacon varieties.

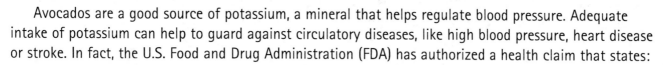

Health Benefits of Avocado

Avocados contain *oleic acid,* a monounsaturated fat that may help to lower cholesterol. In one study of people with moderately high cholesterol levels, individuals who ate a diet high in avocados showed clear health improvements. After seven days on the diet that included avocados, they had significant decreases in total cholesterol and LDL cholesterol, along with an 11% increase in health promoting HDL cholesterol.

Avocados are a good source of potassium, a mineral that helps regulate blood pressure. Adequate intake of potassium can help to guard against circulatory diseases, like high blood pressure, heart disease or stroke. In fact, the U.S. Food and Drug Administration (FDA) has authorized a health claim that states:

> *"Diets containing foods that are good sources of potassium and low in sodium may reduce the risk of high blood pressure and stroke."*

One cup of avocado has 23% of the Daily Value for *folate,* a nutrient important for heart health. To determine the relationship between folate intake and heart disease, researchers followed over 80,000 women for 14 years using dietary questionnaires. They found that women who had higher intakes of dietary folate had a 55% lower risk of having heart attacks or fatal heart disease. Another study showed that individuals who consume folate-rich diets have a much lower risk of cardiovascular disease or stroke than those who do not consume as much of this vital nutrient.

Description of Avocado

The avocado is colloquially known as the Alligator Pear, reflecting its shape and the leather-like appearance of its skin. Avocado is derived from the Aztec word "ahuacatl."

Avocados are the fruit from the *Persea Americana,* a tall evergreen tree that can grow up to 65 feet in height. There are dozens of varieties of avocadoes, which fall into three main categories — Mexican, Guatemalan, and West Indian — which differ in their size, appearance, quality and susceptibility to cold. The most popular type of avocado in the United States is the Haas variety, which has rugged, pebbly brown-black skin. Another common type of avocado is the Fuerte, which is larger than the Haas and has smooth, dark green skin and a more defined pear shape.

Avocados vary in weight from 8 ounces to 3 pounds depending upon the variety. The edible portion of the avocado is its yellow-green flesh, which has a luscious, buttery consistency and a subtle nutty flavor. The skin and pit are inedible.

Heavyweight Healing Foods—CONTINUED

History of the Avocado

Avocados are native to Central and South America and have been cultivated in these regions since 8,000 B.C. In the mid-17th century, they were introduced to Jamaica and spread through the Asian tropical regions in the mid-1800s. Cultivation in the United States, specifically in Florida and California, began in the early 20th century. While avocados are now grown in most tropical and subtropical countries, the major commercial producers include the United States (Florida and California), Mexico, the Dominican Republic, Brazil and Colombia.

How to Select and Store Avocado

A ripe, ready to eat avocado is slightly soft but should have no dark sunken spots or cracks. If the avocado has a slight neck, rather than being rounded on top, it was probably tree ripened and will have better flavor. A firmer, less mature fruit can be ripened at home and will be less likely to have bruises. The Haas avocado weighs about 8 ounces on average and has a pebbled dark green or black skin, while the Fuerte avocado has smoother, brighter green skin. Avoid Fuertes with skin that is too light and bright. Florida avocados, which can be as large as 5 pounds, have less fat and calories, but their taste is not as rich as California varieties.

A firm avocado will ripen in a paper bag or in a fruit basket at room temperature within a few days. As the fruit ripens, the skin will turn darker. Avocados should not be refrigerated until they are ripe. Once ripe, they can be kept refrigerated for up to a week if they have not been sliced.

Safety of Avocados

Avocados contain enzymes called *chitinases* that can cause allergic reactions in people with latex sensitivities. Studies have shown a strong association between latex allergies and allergic reactions to avocado. The treatment of avocados with ethylene gas to induce ripening can increase the presence of these allergenic enzymes. Individuals with latex allergy should avoid eating avocados in cooked or raw form. However, if you really love avocados, some evidence suggests that cooked forms of this food may be acceptable for allergy-sensitive individuals since cooking can deactivate the enzymes that may be responsible for the cross-reaction with latex.

BLUEBERRIES

With flavors that range from mildly sweet to tart and tangy, blueberries are nutritional stars bursting with nutrition and flavor while being very low in calories. Blueberries are at their best from May through October when they are in season.

Blueberries are the fruits of a shrub that belong to the *heath* family, which includes the cranberry and bilberry as well as the azalea, mountain laurel and rhododendron. Blueberries grow in clusters and range in size from that of a small pea to a marble. They are deep in color, ranging from blue to maroon to purple-black, and feature a white-gray waxy "bloom" that covers the surface serving as a protective coat. The skin surrounds a semi-transparent flesh that encases tiny seeds.

Heavyweight Healing Foods—CONTINUED

Health Benefits of Blueberries

Recently, researchers at Tufts University analyzed 60 fruits and vegetables for their antioxidant capability. Blueberries came out on top, rating highest in their capacity to destroy free radicals.

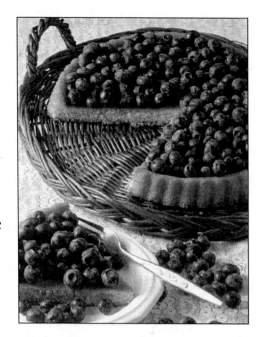

The Blueberry is an Antioxidant Powerhouse

Packed with antioxidant phytonutrients called *anthocyanidins,* blueberries neutralize free-radical damage to the collagen matrix of cells and tissues that can lead to cataracts, glaucoma, varicose veins, hemorrhoids, peptic ulcers, heart disease and cancer. *Anthocyanins,* the blue-red pigments found in blueberries, improve the integrity of support structures in the veins and entire vascular system. Anthocyanins have been shown to enhance the effects of Vitamin C, improve capillary integrity, and stabilize the *collagen matrix* (the ground substance of all body tissues). They work their protective magic by preventing free-radical damage, inhibiting enzymes from cleaving the collagen matrix, and directly cross-linking with collagen fibers to form a more stable collagen matrix.

A Visionary Fruit

Extracts of *bilberry* (a variety of blueberry) have been shown in numerous studies to improve nighttime visual acuity and promote quicker adjustment to darkness and faster restoration of visual acuity after exposure to glare. This research was conducted to evaluate claims of bilberry's beneficial effects on night vision made by British Air Force pilots during World War II who regularly consumed bilberry preserves before their night missions.

A Better Brain with Blueberries

In animal studies, researchers have found that blueberries help protect the brain from oxidative stress and may reduce the effects of age-related conditions such as Alzheimer's disease or dementia. Researchers found that diets rich in blueberries significantly improved both the learning capacity and motor skills of aging rats, making them mentally equivalent to much younger rats.

Healthier Elimination with Blueberries

Blueberries can help relieve both diarrhea and constipation. In addition to soluble and insoluble fiber, blueberries also contain *tannins,* which act as astringents in the digestive system to reduce inflammation. Blueberries also promote urinary tract health. Blueberries contain the same compounds found in cranberries that help prevent or eliminate urinary tract infections. In order for bacteria to infect, they must first adhere to the mucosal lining of the urethra and bladder. Components found in cranberry and blueberry juice reduce the ability of *E. coli,* the bacteria which is the most common cause of urinary tract infections, to adhere.

Heavyweight Healing Foods—CONTINUED

History of Blueberries

Blueberries are native to North America where they grow throughout the woods and mountainous regions in the United States and Canada. This fruit is rarely found growing in Europe and has only been recently introduced in Australia.

There are approximately 30 different species of blueberries with different ones growing throughout various regions. For example, the Highbush variety can be found throughout the Eastern seaboard from Maine to Florida, the Lowbush variety throughout the Northeast and Eastern Canada, and the Evergreen variety throughout states in the Pacific Northwest.

While blueberries played an important role in North American Indian food culture, being an ingredient in *pemmican,* a traditional dish composed of the fruit and dried meat, they were not consumed in great amounts by the colonists until the mid-19th century. This seems to be related to the fact that people did not appreciate their tart flavor, and only when sugar became more widely available as a sweetener at this time, did they become more popular.

Blueberries were not cultivated until the beginning of the 20th century, becoming commercially available in 1916. Cultivation of blueberries was spearheaded by a botanist at the USDA who pioneered research into blueberry production. His work was continued by Elizabeth White, whose family established the first commercial blueberry fields.

How to Select and Store Blueberries

Choose blueberries that are firm and have a lively, uniform hue colored with a whitish bloom. Shake the container, noticing whether berries have the tendency to move freely; if they do not, this may indicate that they are soft and damaged or moldy. Avoid berries that appear dull in color or are soft and watery in texture. They should be free from moisture since the presence of water will cause the berries to decay. When purchasing frozen berries, shake the bag gently to ensure that the berries move freely and are not clumped together, which may suggest that they have been thawed and refrozen. Blueberries that are cultivated in the United States are available from May through October while imported berries may be found at other times of the year.

Ripe blueberries should be stored in a covered container in the refrigerator where they will keep for about a week, although they will be freshest if consumed within a few days. Always check berries before storing and remove any damaged berries to prevent the spread of mold. But don't wash berries until right before eating, as washing will remove the bloom that protects the fruit's skin from degradation. If kept out at room temperature for more than a day, the berries may spoil.

Ripe berries can also be frozen, although this will slightly change their texture and flavor. Before freezing, wash, drain and remove any damaged berries. To better ensure uniform texture upon thawing, spread the berries out on a cookie sheet or baking pan, place in the freezer until frozen, then put the berries in a plastic bag for storage in the freezer. Berries should last up to a year in the freezer.

Heavyweight Healing Foods—CONTINUED

Safety of Blueberries

Blueberries are among a small number of foods that contain a measurable amount of *oxalates,* naturally occurring substances found in plants, animals, and human beings. When oxalates become too concentrated in body fluids, they can crystallize and cause health problems. For this reason, individuals with already existing and untreated kidney or gallbladder problems may want to avoid eating large amounts of blueberries. Oxalates may also interfere with absorption of calcium from the body. For this reason, individuals trying to increase their calcium stores may want to avoid eating blueberries with calcium-rich foods, or if taking calcium supplements, may want to eat them 2-3 hours before or after taking their supplements.

BROCCOLI

The hearty structure, fresh appearance and ease of preparation combined with its exceptional nutritional value help to make broccoli one of the favorite vegetables of health conscious American consumers. While it is available year-round, the season for broccoli runs from October through May when it has the best flavor and is of the highest quality.

Broccoli is a member of the cabbage family, and is closely related to cauliflower. Its cultivation originated in Italy. *Broccolo,* its Italian name, means "cabbage sprout." Because of its different components, broccoli provides a range of tastes and textures, from soft and flowery (the floret) to fibrous and crunchy (the stem and stalk).

Do not let the smell of the sulfur compounds that are released while cooking keep you away from these highly nutritious vegetables!

Cancer Protective Benefits of Broccoli

Like other cruciferous vegetables, broccoli contains phytochemicals — *sulforaphane* and the *indoles* — with significant anti-cancer effects. Research on *indole-3-carbinol* shows this compound helps deactivate a potent estrogen metabolite (2-hydroxyestrone) that promotes tumor growth, especially in estrogen-sensitive breast cells. Indole-3-carbinol has been shown to suppress not only breast tumor cell growth, but also cancer cell *metastasis* (the movement of cancerous cells to other parts of the body). Scientists have found that sulforaphane boosts the body's detoxification enzymes, potentially by altering gene expression, thus helping to clear potentially carcinogenic substances more quickly. When researchers at Johns Hopkins studied the effect of sulphoraphane on tumor formation in lab animals, those animals given sulforaphane had fewer tumors, and the tumors they did develop grew more slowly and weighed less, meaning they were smaller.

A study published in the cancer journal, *Oncology Report* demonstrated that sulforaphane, which is a potent inducer of Phase 2 liver detoxification enzymes, also has a dose-dependent ability to induce cell growth arrest and cell death via *apoptosis* (the self-destruct sequence the body uses to eliminate abnormal cells) in both leukemia and melanoma cells.

Heavyweight Healing Foods—CONTINUED

Now, a new study published in the *Journal of Nutrition* shows sulforaphane also helps stop the proliferation of breast cancer cells, even in the later stages of their growth. If broccoli isn't one of your favorite vegetables, remember that a tablespoon of broccoli sprouts contains as much sulforaphane as is found in a whole pound of adult broccoli.

Broccoli definitely proves the adage, "Good things come in small packages." Broccoli sprouts concentrate phytochemicals found in mature broccoli — a lot. Researchers estimate that broccoli sprouts contain 10-100 times the power of mature broccoli to boost enzymes that detoxify potential carcinogens! A healthy serving of broccoli sprouts in your salad or sandwich can offer as much or even more protection against cancer as larger amounts of mature broccoli.

Description of Broccoli

Broccoli's name is derived from the Latin word *brachium,* which means branch or arm, a reflection of its tree-like shape that features a compact head of florets attached by small stems to a larger stalk. Its color can range from deep sage to dark green to purplish-green, depending upon the variety. The most popular type of broccoli sold in the United States is known as Italian green, or *Calabrese,* named after the Italian province of Calabria where it first grew. Other vegetables related to broccoli are *broccolini,* a mix between broccoli and kale, and *broccoflower,* a cross between broccoli and cauliflower.

History of Broccoli

Broccoli has its roots in Italy in ancient Roman times when it was developed from wild cabbage, a plant that more resembles collards than broccoli. It spread throughout the Near East where it was appreciated for its edible flower heads and was subsequently brought back to Italy where it was further cultivated. Broccoli was introduced to the United States in colonial times, popularized by Italian immigrants who brought this prized vegetable with them to the New World.

How to Select and Store Broccoli

Choose broccoli with floret clusters that are compact and not bruised. They should be uniformly colored, either dark green, sage or purple-green, depending upon variety, and with no yellowing. In addition, they should not have any yellow flowers blossoming through, as this is a sign of over maturity. The stalk and stems should be firm, yet tender with no slimy spots appearing either there or on the florets. If leaves are attached, they should be vibrant in color and not wilted.

Broccoli is very perishable and should be stored in an open plastic bag in the refrigerator crisper where it will keep for about four days. Since water on the surface will encourage its degradation, do not wash the broccoli before refrigerating. Broccoli that has been blanched and then frozen can stay up to a year. Leftover cooked broccoli should be placed in tightly covered container and stored in the refrigerator where it will keep for a few days.

Safety of Broccoli

Broccoli contains *goitrogens,* naturally occurring substances in certain foods that can interfere with the functioning of the thyroid gland. Individuals with already existing and untreated thyroid problems may

Heavyweight Healing Foods—CONTINUED

want to avoid broccoli for this reason. Cooking may help to inactivate the goitrogenic compounds found in food. However, it is not clear from the research exactly what percent of goitrogenic compounds get inactivated by cooking, or exactly how much risk is involved with the consumption of broccoli by individuals with pre-existing and untreated thyroid problems.

EGGS, HEN

The incredible and edible egg is available year round to provide not only delicious meals on their own but an essential ingredient for the many baked goods and sauces that would never be the same without them.

Composed of a yellow yolk and translucent white surrounded by a protective shell, the incredible nature of the egg is partially found in their unique food chemistry which allows them help in coagulation, foaming, emulsification and browning.

Health Benefits of Eggs

Eggs are a good source of low-cost high-quality protein, providing 5.5 grams of protein (11.1% of the daily value for protein) in one egg for a caloric cost of only 68 calories. The structure of humans and animals is built on protein. We rely on animal and vegetable protein for our supply of amino acids, and then our bodies rearrange the nitrogen to create the pattern of amino acids we require.

Another health benefit of eggs is their contribution to the diet as a source of choline. Although our bodies can produce some choline, we cannot make enough to make up for an inadequate supply in our diets, and choline deficiency can also cause deficiency of another B vitamin critically important for health, folic acid.

Researchers at the U.S. Department of Agriculture conducted a study to see what would happen if human subjects received a diet low in choline and folate. Male and female volunteers ate low-choline, low-folate meals that provided as little as 13% of the recommended daily allowance of folate. No severe choline or folate deficiencies occurred during the study, but blood levels of choline decreased an average of 25–28% in men and women during the low-choline, low-folate regimes. Levels returned to at least normal when researchers provided more of these important B vitamins to the people in the tests.

Choline is definitely a nutrient needed in good supply for good health. Choline is a key component of many fat-containing structures in cell membranes, whose flexibility and integrity depend on adequate supplies of choline. Two fat-like molecules in the brain, *phosphatidylcholine* and *sphingomyelin,* account for an unusually high percentage of the brain's total mass, so choline is particularly important for brain function and health.

In addition, choline is a highly important molecule in a cellular process called *methylation.* Many important chemical events in the body are made possible by methylation, in which methyl groups are transferred from one place to another. For example, genes in the body can be switched on or turned off in this way, and cells use methylation to send messages back and forth. Choline, which contains three methyl groups, is highly active in this process.

Heavyweight Healing Foods—CONTINUED

Choline is also a key component of acetylcholine. A neurotrasmitter that carries messages to and from nerves, acetylcholine is the body's primary chemical means of sending messages between nerves and muscles.

One large egg provides 300 micrograms of choline (all in the yolk), and also contains 315 milligrams (yes, milligrams not micrograms) of phosphatidylcholine. Although most sources just report the free choline at 300 micrograms, it is the phosphatidylcholine that is the most common form in which choline is incorporated into cell membrane phospholipids.

In addition to its significant effects on brain function and the nervous system, choline also has an impact on cardiovascular health since it is one of the B vitamins that helps convert *homocysteine,* a molecule that can damage blood vessels, into other benign substances. Eggs are also a good source of Vitamin B12, another B vitamin that is of major importance in the process of converting homocysteine into safe molecules. Eggs are high in cholesterol, and health experts in the past, counseled people to therefore avoid this food. (All of the cholesterol in the egg is in the yolk.) However, nutrition experts have now determined people on a low-fat diet can eat one or two eggs a day without measurable changes in their blood cholesterol levels. This information is supported by a statistical analysis of 224 dietary studies carried out over the past 25 years that investigated the relationship between diet and blood cholesterol levels in over 8,000 subjects. What investigators in this study found was that saturated fat in the diet, not dietary cholesterol, is what influences blood cholesterol levels the most.

Improve Your Cholesterol Profile With Eggs

Not only have studies shown that eggs do not significantly affect cholesterol levels in most individuals, but the latest research suggests that eating whole eggs may actually result in significant improvement in one's blood *lipids* (cholesterol) profile — even in persons whose cholesterol levels rise when eating cholesterol-rich foods.

In northern Mexico, an area in which the diet contains a high amount of fat because of its reliance on low-cost meat products and tortillas made with hydrogenated oils, coronary artery disease is common. In a study published in the *American Journal of Clinical Nutrition,* researchers evaluated the effects of daily consumption of whole eggs on the ratio of LDL (bad) cholesterol to HDL (good) cholesterol, and *phenotype* (the way an individual's genetic possibilities are actually expressed) in 54 children (8-12 years old) from this region. A month of eating 2 eggs daily, not only did not worsen the children's ratio of LDL:HDL, which remained the same, but the size of their LDL cholesterol increased — a very beneficial change since larger LDL is much less *atherogenic* (likely to promote atherosclerosis) than the smaller LDL subfractions. Among children who originally had the high risk LDL phenotype B, 15% shifted to the low-risk LDL phenotype A after just one month of eating whole eggs.

Description of Eggs

Eggs are *egg-ceptional* foods. They are whole foods, prepackaged sources of carbohydrates, protein, fat and micronutrients. Yet, their *eggs-quisite* nutritional value should not be surprising when you remember that an egg contains everything needed for the nourishment of a developing chick. In Latin, the scientific name for chicken is *Gallus domesticus.*

Heavyweight Healing Foods—CONTINUED

Eggs are composed of a yellow yolk and translucent white surrounded by a protective shell that can be white or brown, depending upon the breed of the chicken. The shell's color is not related to the quality or nutritional value of the egg itself.

In addition to their wonderful taste and nutritional content, eggs hold an esteemed place in cooking since due to their food chemistry, they serve many unique functions in recipes, including coagulation, foaming, emulsification and browning.

History of Eggs

The history of the egg as food runs mostly parallel with the history of people consuming chicken as food. Although it is uncertain when and where it began, the practice of raising chickens for food is ancient and so, subsequently, is the consumption of eggs as food, extending back to the times of early man.

Eggs have always been a symbol of fertility and have been an icon of religious worship. To this day, there is folklore surrounding eggs that is enjoyed by different cultures around the world. One of the most widely held food and holiday associations is that of the Easter egg. How the egg became associated with this holiday seems to have roots that are both biological and cultural. Before more modern techniques of poultry raising, hens laid few eggs during the winter. This meant that Easter, occurring with the advent of Spring, coincided with the hen's renewed cycle of laying numerous eggs. Additionally, since eggs were traditionally considered a food of luxury, they were forbidden during Lent, so Christians had to wait until Easter to eat them — another reason eggs became associated with this holiday. Interestingly enough, the custom of painting eggshells has an extensive history and was a popular custom among many ancient civilizations, including the Egyptians, Chinese, Greeks and Persians.

How to Select and Store Eggs

Often, eggs are classified according to the USDA grading system and bear a label of AA, A, or B. This grading is an indicator of quality parameters, including freshness, with AA being of the most superior in quality. Eggs are also labeled according to their size — extra large, large, medium and small — which is graded according to a standard.

Yet, you may not see any labeling on the eggs you buy since it is not legally mandatory that they be inspected and graded by these federal standards. This is often the situation when you buy farm fresh eggs from a local purveyor. If this is the case, get to know the seller and his or her reputation and make sure that, as usual, the eggs are kept refrigerated. Inspect any eggs that you purchase for breaks or cracks. And of course, take care when packing them in your shopping bag for the trip home, as they are very fragile.

Store eggs in the refrigerator where they will stay fresh for about one month. Do not wash them as this can remove their protective coating. Keep them in their original carton or in a covered container so that they do not absorb odors or lose any moisture. Do not store them in the refrigerator door since this exposes them to too much heat each time the refrigerator is opened and closed. Make sure to store them with their pointed end facing downward as this will help to prevent the air chamber, and the yolk, from being displaced.

Heavyweight Healing Foods—CONTINUED

Safe Handling of Eggs

Health safety concerns about eggs center on *salmonellosis* (salmonella-caused food poisoning). Salmonella bacteria from the chicken's intestines may be found even in clean, un-cracked eggs. Formerly, these bacteria were found only in eggs with cracked shells. Safe food techniques, like washing the eggs before cracking them, may not protect you from infection. To destroy the bacteria, eggs must be cooked at high enough temperatures for a sufficient length of time to destroy the bacteria. Soft-cooked, sunny-side up or raw eggs carry salmonellosis risk. Hard-boiled, scrambled, or poached eggs do not.

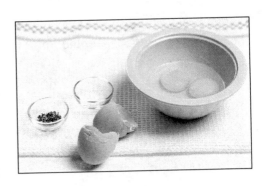

Dishes and utensils used when preparing eggs should be washed in warm water separately from other kitchenware, and hand washing with warm, soapy water is essential after handling eggs. Any surfaces that might have potentially come into contact with raw egg should be washed and can be sanitized with a solution of 1 teaspoon chlorine to 1 quart water.

Egg and Food Allergy

Although allergic reactions can occur to virtually any food, research studies on food allergy consistently report more problems with some foods than with others. Common symptoms associated with an allergic reaction to food include:

- Chronic gastrointestinal disturbances
- Frequent ear and bladder infections
- Bed-wetting
- Asthma and sinusitis
- Eczema, skin rashes, acne, and hives
- Bursitis and joint pain

- Fatigue
- Headaches and migraines
- Hyperactivity
- Depression
- Insomnia

Individuals who suspect food allergy to be an underlying factor in their health problems may want to avoid commonly allergenic foods. Eggs are one of the foods most commonly associated with allergic reactions. Other foods commonly associated with allergic reactions include:

- Cow's milk
- Wheat
- Beef
- Soybeans
- Oranges

- Corn
- Pork
- Chicken
- Peanuts

- Yeast
- Strawberry
- Tomato
- Spinach

These foods do not need to be eaten in their pure, isolated form in order to trigger an adverse reaction. For example, yogurt made from cow's milk is also a common allergenic food, even though the cow's milk has been processed and fermented in order to make the yogurt. Ice cream made from cow's milk would be an equally good example.

Heavyweight Healing Foods—CONTINUED

FLAX SEEDS

The warm, earthy and subtly nutty flavor of flax seeds combined with an abundance of Omega-3 fatty acids makes them an increasingly popular addition to the diets of many a health conscious consumer. Whole and ground seeds and oils are available throughout the year; it is recommended to purchase refrigerated packages of ground flax seeds and oil because they can spoil easily.

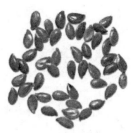

Flax seeds are slightly larger than sesame seeds and have a hard shell that is smooth and shiny. Their color ranges from deep amber to reddish brown depending upon whether the flax is of the golden or brown variety.

Health Benefits of Flax Seed

Flax seed oil is rich in alpha linolenic acid, an Omega-3 fat that is a precursor to the form of Omega-3 found in fish oils called *eicosapentaenoic acid* (EPA). *Alpha linolenic acid* (ALA), in addition to providing several beneficial effects of its own, can be converted in the body to EPA, thus providing EPA's beneficial effects. For this conversion to readily take place, however, depends on the presence and activity of an enzyme called *delta-6-destaurase*, which, in some individuals, is less available or less active than in others. In addition, delta-6-desaturase function is inhibited in diabetes and by the consumption of saturated fat and alcohol. For these reasons, higher amounts of ALA-rich flax seed oil must be consumed to provide the same benefits as the Omega-3 fats found in the oil of cold-water fish.

A recent MedLine check (MedLine provides access to the published peer-reviewed medical literature) revealed 1,677 research articles on linolenic acid, investigating its effects on numerous physiological processes and health conditions.

Anti-Inflammatory Benefits of Flax Seed

Omega-3 fats are used by the body to produce Series 1 and 3 prostaglandins, which are anti-inflammatory hormone-like molecules, in contrast to the Series 2 prostaglandins, which are pro-inflammatory molecules produced from other fats, notably the Omega-6 fats, which are found in high amounts in animal fats, margarine, and many vegetable oils including corn, safflower, sunflower, palm, and peanut oils. Omega-3 fats can help reduce the inflammation that is a significant factor in conditions such as asthma, osteoarthritis, rheumatoid arthritis, and migraine headaches.

Flax Seed is Rich in Beneficial Fiber

Flax seeds' Omega-3 fats are far from all this exceptional food has to offer. Flax seed meal and flour provides a very good source of fiber that can lower cholesterol levels in people with atherosclerosis and diabetic heart disease, reduce the exposure of colon cells to cancer-causing chemicals, relieve the constipation or diarrhea of irritable bowel syndrome sufferers, and help stabilize blood sugar levels in diabetic patients. Flax seeds are also a good source of magnesium, which helps to reduce the severity of asthma by keeping airways relaxed and open, lowers high blood pressure and reduces the risk of heart attack and stroke in people with atherosclerosis and diabetic heart disease, prevents the blood vessel spasm that leads to migraine attacks, and generally promotes relaxation and restores normal sleep patterns.

Heavyweight Healing Foods—CONTINUED

A study published in the *Archives of Internal Medicine* confirms that eating high fiber foods, such as flax seed, helps prevent heart disease. Almost 10,000 American adults participated in this study and were followed for 19 years, during which time 1,843 cases of *coronary heart disease* (CHD) and 3,762 cases of *cardiovascular disease* (CVD) were diagnosed. People eating the most fiber, 21 grams per day, had 12% less CHD and 11% less CVD compared to those eating the least, 5 grams daily. Those eating the most water-soluble dietary fiber fared even better with a 15% reduction in risk of CHD and a 10% risk reduction in CVD without breast cancer. In animal studies conducted to evaluate lignans' beneficial effect, supplementing a high-fat diet with flax seed flour reduced early markers for mammary cancer in rats by more than 55%.

Description of Flax Seed

What's in a name? Well, when it comes to the scientific name of flax seeds, the name says it all. Flax seeds are known as *Linum usitatissimum* with it species name meaning "most useful." That would definitely describe the versatility and nutritional value of this tiny little seed.

Their flavor is warm and earthy with a subtly nutty edge. While whole flax seeds feature a soft crunch, they are usually not consumed whole but rather ground since this allows for the enhancement of their nutrient absorption. Ground flax seeds can have a relatively mealy texture with a potential hint of crunch depending upon how fine they are ground.

History of Flax Seed

Flax seeds have a long and extensive history. Originating in Mesopotamia, the flax plant has been known since the Stone Ages. One of the first records of the culinary use of flax seeds is from times of ancient Greece. In both that civilization and in ancient Rome, the health benefits of flax seeds were widely praised. After the fall of Rome, the cultivation and popularity of flax seeds declined.

Ironically, it was Charlemagne, the emperor who would be famous for shaping European history, who also helped to shape the history of flax seeds, restoring them to their noble position in the food culture of Europe. Charlemagne was impressed with how useful flax was in terms of its culinary, medicinal, and fiber usefulness (flax seed fibers can be woven into linen) that he passed laws requiring not only its cultivation but its consumption as well. After Charlemange, flax seeds became widely appreciated throughout Europe.

It was not until the early colonists arrived in North America that flax was first planted in the United States. In the 17th century, flax was first introduced and planted in Canada, the country that is currently the major producer of this extremely beneficial seed.

How to Select and Store Flax Seed

Flax seeds can be purchased either whole or already ground. The two different forms offer distinct benefits. Although ground flax seeds may be more convenient, whole flax seeds feature a longer shelf life.

Whole flax seeds are generally available in prepackaged containers as well as bulk bins. Just as with any other food that you may purchase in the bulk section, make sure that the bins containing the flax seeds are covered and that the store has a good product turnover so as to ensure their maximal freshness.

Heavyweight Healing Foods—CONTINUED

Whether purchasing flax seeds in bulk or in a packaged container, make sure that there is no evidence of moisture. If you purchase whole flax seeds, store them in an airtight container in a dark, dry and cool place where they will keep fresh for several months.

Ground flax seeds are usually available both refrigerated and non-refrigerated. It is highly recommended to purchase ground flax seed that is in a vacuum-sealed package or has been refrigerated since once flax seeds are ground, they are much more prone to oxidation and spoilage. Likewise, if you either purchase ground flax seeds or you grind them at home, it is important to keep them in a tightly sealed container in the refrigerator or freezer to prevent them from becoming rancid.

Flax seed oil is especially perishable and should be purchased in opaque bottles that have been kept refrigerated. Flax seed oil should have a sweet nutty flavor. Never use flax seed oil in cooking; add it to foods after they have been heated.

Safety of Flax Seed

Flax seeds are not a commonly allergenic food, are not included in the list of 20 foods that most frequently contain pesticide residues, and are also not known to contain goitrogens, oxalates, or purines.

LEMON AND LIMES

Although lemons and limes may not be what you would choose for an afternoon snack, we consider them as powerhouses when we want to bring out the flavor of other foods. While both are available throughout the year, lemons are in the peak of their season around May, June and August while limes are at their peak from May through October.

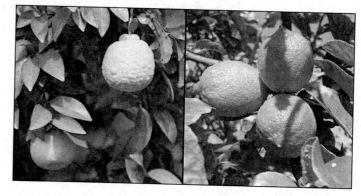

Lemons are oval in shape and feature a yellow, textured outer peel. Like other citrus fruits, their inner flesh is encased in eight to ten segments.

Usually smaller than lemons, limes are oval or round in shape having a diameter of one to two inches with green flesh and skin. They can be either sour or sweet depending on the variety; however, sweet limes are not readily available in the United States. Sour limes contain citric acid giving them an acidic and tart taste, while sweet limes lack citric acid and are sweeter in flavor.

Lemons Provide Phytonutrients with Antioxidant, Anti-Cancer and Antibiotic Effects

Like many of the fruits and vegetables found in the world's healthiest foods, lemons and limes contain unique flavonoid compounds that have antioxidant and anti-cancer properties. Of special interest in limes have been flavonoids called *flavonol glycosides*, including many *kaempferol*-related molecules. While these flavonoids have been shown to stop cell division in many cancer cell lines, they are perhaps most interesting for their antibiotic effects. In several villages in West Africa where cholera epidemics had occurred, the

Heavyweight Healing Foods—CONTINUED

inclusion of lime juice during the main meal of the day was determined to have been protective against the contraction of cholera. (Cholera is a disease triggered by activity of the bacteria called *Vibrio cholera*.) Researchers quickly began to experiment with the addition of lime juice to the sauce eaten with rice, and in this role, lime juice was also found to have a strong protective effect against cholera.

Several other fascinating research studies on the healing properties of lemons and limes have shown that cell cycles — including the decision a cell makes about whether to divide (called *mitosis*) or die (*apoptosis*) — are altered by lime juice, as are the activities of special immune cells called *monocytes*.

In addition to their unique phytonutrient properties, lemons and limes are an excellent source of one of the most important antioxidants in nature, Vitamin C. Vitamin C is one of the main antioxidants found in food and the primary water-soluble antioxidant in the body. Vitamin C travels through the body neutralizing any free-radicals with which it comes into contact in the aqueous environments in the body both inside and outside cells. Free-radicals can interact with the healthy cells of the body, damaging them and their membranes, and also cause a lot of inflammation, or painful swelling, in the body. This is one of the reasons that Vitamin C has been shown to be helpful for reducing some of the symptoms of osteoarthritis and rheumatoid arthritis.

Since free-radicals can damage blood vessels and can change cholesterol to make it more likely to build up in artery walls, Vitamin C can be helpful for preventing the development and progression of atherosclerosis and diabetic heart disease.

Vitamin C is also vital to the function of a strong immune system. The immune system's main goal is to protect you from illness, so a little extra Vitamin C may be useful in conditions like colds, flu's, and recurrent ear infections. Owing to the multitude of Vitamin C's health benefits, it is not surprising that research has shown that consumption of vegetables and fruits high in this nutrient is associated with a reduced risk of death from all causes including heart disease, stroke and cancer.

Description of Lemons

Lemons, scientifically known as *Citrus limon,* are more commonly known as the fruit that evokes images of sunshine and the sweet smiles of children standing roadside at their homemade lemonade stands.

While most lemons are tart, acidic and astringent, they are also surprisingly refreshing. The two main types of sour lemons are the Eureka and the Lisbon. The Eureka generally has more textured skin, a short neck at one end and a few seeds, while the Lisbon has smoother skin, no neck and is generally seedless. In addition to these sour lemons, there are also some varieties that are sweet in flavor. One notable example is the Meyer lemon that is becoming more popular in both markets and restaurants.

Heavyweight Healing Foods—CONTINUED

Description of Limes

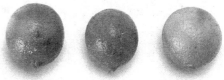

Limes are a small citrus fruit, *Citrus aurantifolia,* whose skin and flesh are green in color and which have an oval or round shape with a diameter between one to two inches. Sour limes possess a greater sugar and citric acid content than lemons and feature an acidic and tart taste, while sweet limes, which lack citric acid content, are sweet in flavor.

There are two general varieties of sour limes available, the Tahitian and the Key. Among Tahitian limes are the egg-shaped Persian and the smaller, seedless Bears. Key limes, famous for the pie bearing their name, are smaller and more acidic than the Tahitian variety.

History of Lemons

Lemons were originally developed as a cross between the lime and the *citron* and are thought to have originated in China or India, having been cultivated in these regions for about 2,500 years. Their first introduction to Europe was by Arabs who brought them to Spain in the 11th century around the same time that they were introduced into Northern Africa. The Crusaders, who found the fruit growing in Palestine, are credited with bringing the lemon to other countries across Europe. Like many other fruits and vegetables, lemons were brought to the Americas by Christopher Columbus in his second voyage to the New World in 1493, and have been grown in Florida since the 16th century.

Lemons, like other Vitamin-C rich fruits, were highly prized by the miners and developers during the California Gold Rush in the mid-19th century, since they were used to protect against the development of *scurvy.* They were in such demand that people were willing to pay up to $1 per lemon, a price that would still be considered costly today and was extremely expensive back in 1849. The major producers of lemons today are the United States and Italy as well as Spain, Greece, Israel and Turkey.

History of Limes

Limes are grown on trees that flourish in tropical and subtropical climates. They were thought to originate in Southeast Asia. Arab traders brought lime trees back from their journey to Asia and introduced them into Egypt and Northern Africa around the 10th century. The Arabian Moors brought them to Spain in the 13th century and then, like many fruits, they were spread throughout southern Europe during the Crusades.

Limes made their way to the New World with Columbus on his second voyage in 1493, and were subsequently planted in many Caribbean countries whose hot, humid climates supported the cultivation of this fruit. Centuries later, British explorers and traders, who were readily using the Vitamin C-rich limes that grew in their West Indies colonies to prevent *scurvy,* earned the nickname "limey," a word that is often still used colloquially for persons of British descent.

The introduction of limes to the United States began in the 16th century when Spanish Explorers brought the West Indies lime to the Florida Keys, beginning the advent of Key limes. In the following century, Spanish missionaries attempted to plant lime trees in California, but the climate did not support their

Heavyweight Healing Foods—CONTINUED

growth. In great demand by the miners and explorers during the California Gold Rush as a fruit that was known to prevent scurvy, limes began to be imported from Tahiti and Mexico at this time in the mid-19th century. Today, Brazil, Mexico and the United States are among the leading commercial producers of limes.

How to Select and Store Lemons

One of the tricks to finding a good quality lemon is to find one that is rather thin-skinned since those with thicker peels will have less flesh and therefore be less juicy. Therefore, choose lemons that are heavy for their size and that feature peels that have a finely grained texture. They should be fully yellow in color as those that have green tinges will be more acidic due to the fact that they have not fully ripened. Signs of over mature fruit include wrinkling, soft or hard patches and dull coloring. Fresh lemons are generally available all year round.

Lemons will stay fresh kept at room temperature, away from exposure to sunlight, for about one week. If you will not be using them within this time period, you can store the lemons in the refrigerator crisper where they will keep for about four weeks.

Lemon juice and zest can also be stored for later use. Place freshly squeezed lemon juice in ice cube trays until frozen, subsequently storing them in plastic bags in the freezer. Dried lemon zest should be stored in a cool and dry place in an airtight glass container.

How to Select and Store Limes

Choose limes that are firm and heavy for their size, free of decay and mold. They should have a glossy skin that is deep green in color; although limes turn more yellow as they ripen, they are at the height of their lively, tart flavor when they are green in color. While brown spots on the skin of limes may not affect their color, limes that are mostly brownish in color should be avoided since this may be an indication that they have "scald" which may cause them to have an undesirable moldy taste. Limes are available in the marketplace throughout the year, although they are usually in greater supply from mid-spring through mid-fall.

Limes can be kept out at room temperature where they will stay fresh for up to one week. Make sure to keep them away from sunlight exposure since it will cause them to turn yellow and will alter their flavor. Limes can be stored in the refrigerator crisper, wrapped in a loosely sealed plastic bag, where they will keep fresh for about 10-14 days. While they can be kept longer than that, for another several weeks, they will begin to lose their characteristic flavor.

Lime juice and zest can also be stored for later use. Place freshly squeezed lime juice in ice cube trays until frozen, subsequently storing them in plastic bags in the freezer. Dried lime zest should be stored in a cool and dry place in an airtight glass container.

Safety of Lemons and Limes

Lemons and limes are not commonly allergenic foods, are not included in the list of 20 foods that most frequently contain pesticide residues, and are also not known to contain *goitrogens, oxalates,* or *purines.*

Heavyweight Healing Foods—CONTINUED

QUINOA

Although not a common item in most kitchens today, quinoa is an amino acid-rich (protein) seed that has a fluffy, creamy, slightly crunchy texture and a somewhat nutty flavor when cooked. Quinoa is available in your local health food stores throughout the year.

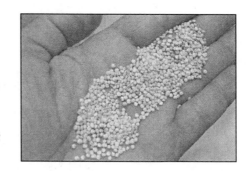

Most commonly considered a grain, quinoa is actually a relative of leafy green vegetables like spinach and Swiss chard.

Health Benefits of Quinoa

A recently rediscovered ancient "grain" native to Central America, quinoa was once called "the gold of the Aztecs," who recognized its value in increasing the stamina of their warriors. Not only is quinoa high in protein, but the protein it supplies is complete protein, meaning that it includes all nine essential amino acids. Not only is quinoa's amino acid profile well balanced, making it a good choice for vegans concerned about adequate protein intake, but quinoa is rich in the amino acid *lysine*, which is essential for tissue growth and repair. In addition to protein, quinoa features a host of other health-building nutrients. Because quinoa is a very good source of manganese as well as a good source of magnesium, iron, copper and phosphorous, this "grain" may be especially valuable for persons with migraine headaches, diabetes and atherosclerosis.

Quinoa Helps Migraine Headaches

If you are prone to migraines, try adding quinoa to your diet. Quinoa is a good source of magnesium, a mineral that helps relax blood vessels, preventing the constriction and rebound dilation characteristic of migraines. Increased intake of magnesium has shown relation to a reduced frequency of headache episodes reported by migraine sufferers. Quinoa is also a good source of riboflavin, which is necessary for proper energy production within cells. *Riboflavin* (also called Vitamin B2) has been shown to help reduce the frequency of attacks in migraine sufferers, most likely by improving the energy metabolism within their brain and muscle cells.

Cardiovascular Benefits of Quinoa

Quinoa is a very good source of magnesium, the mineral that relaxes blood vessels. Since low dietary levels of magnesium are associated with increased rates of hypertension, ischemic heart disease and heart arrhythmias, this ancient grain can offer yet another way to provide cardiovascular health for those concerned about atherosclerosis.

Antioxidant Protection of Quinoa

Quinoa is a very good source of manganese and a good source of copper, two minerals that serve as cofactors for the *superoxide dismutase enzyme*. Superoxide dismutase is an antioxidant that helps to protect the mitochondria from oxidative damage created during energy production and guards other cells, such as red blood cells, from injury caused by free-radicals.

Heavyweight Healing Foods—CONTINUED

Description of Quinoa

We usually think of quinoa as a grain, but it is actually the seed of a plant that, as its scientific name *Chenopodium quinoa* reflects, is related to beets, chard and spinach. These amino acid-rich seeds are not only very nutritious, but also very delicious. While the most popular type of quinoa is a transparent yellow color, other varieties feature colors such as orange, pink, red, purple or black. Although often difficult to find in the marketplace, the leaves of the quinoa plant are edible, with a taste similar to its green-leafed relatives, spinach, chard and beets.

History of Quinoa

While relatively new to the United States, quinoa has been cultivated in the Andean mountain regions of Peru, Chile and Bolivia for over 5,000 years, and it has long been a staple food in the diets of the native Indians. The Incas considered it a sacred food and referred to it as the "mother seed."

In their attempts to destroy and control the South American Indians and their culture, the Spanish conquerors destroyed the fields in which quinoa was grown. They made it illegal for the Indians to grow quinoa, with punishment including sentencing the offenders to death. With these harsh measures, the cultivation of quinoa was all but extinguished.

Yet, this super food would not be extinguished forever. In the 1980s, two Americans, discovering the concentrated nutrition potential of quinoa, began cultivating it in Colorado. Since then, quinoa has become more and more available as people realize that it is an exceptionally beneficial food.

How to Select and Store Quinoa

Quinoa is generally available in prepackaged containers as well as bulk bins. Just as with any other food that you may purchase in the bulk section, make sure that the bins containing the quinoa are covered and that the store has a good product turnover so as to ensure its maximal freshness. Whether purchasing quinoa in bulk or in a packaged container, make sure that there is no evidence of moisture. Store quinoa in an airtight container. It will keep for a longer period of time, approximately three to six months, if stored in the refrigerator.

When deciding upon the amount to purchase, remember that quinoa expands during the cooking process to several times its original size. If you cannot find it in your local supermarket, look for it at natural foods stores, which usually carry this super grain.

Safety of Quinoa

This food is not a commonly allergenic food, is not included in the list of 20 foods that most frequently contain pesticide residues, and is also not known to contain *goitrogens, oxalates,* or *purines.*

Heavyweight Healing Foods—CONTINUED

SALMON

Delicious with exceptional nutritional value found in few other foods (Omega-3 fatty acids), the lovely pink-hued salmon can be served in a variety of ways and is always a favorite among fish lovers and enjoyed even by those who are not always fond of fish. The season for the different species of salmon ranges from early summer to late fall, however, the increased production of farm-raised salmon has made it available fresh in local supermarkets year round.

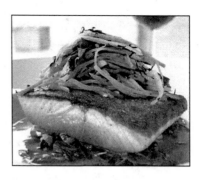

Salmon are incredible fish traveling thousands of miles throughout their life cycle and within two to five years returning to the very location where they were born to spawn and die. The specific characteristics and life cycles of salmon vary with each species. Their flesh ranges in color from pink to red to orange with some varieties richer in important Omega-3 fatty acids than others. For example, chinook and sockeye have more fat than pink and chum and contain great amounts of healthy Omega-3 fatty acids.

Health Benefits of Salmon

Salmon is low in calories and saturated fat, yet high in protein, and a unique type of health-promoting fat, the Omega-3 essential fatty acids. As their name implies, essential fatty acids are essential for human health but because they are not made by the body, they must be obtained from foods. Fish contains a type of essential fatty acid called the Omega-3 fatty acids. Wild-caught cold-water fish, like salmon, are higher in Omega-3 fatty acids than warm water fish. In addition to being an excellent source of Omega-3s, salmon is an excellent source of *selenium,* a very good source of protein, niacin and Vitamin B12, and a good source of phosphorous, magnesium and Vitamin B6.

Cardiovascular Benefits of Salmon

The Omega-3 fats found in salmon have a broad array of beneficial cardiovascular effects. Omega-3s help prevent erratic heart rhythms, make blood less likely to clot inside arteries (the proximate cause of most heart attacks), improve the ratio of good cholesterol to bad cholesterol, and prevent cholesterol from becoming damaged. (Only after cholesterol has been damaged does it clog arteries.)

Omega-3s work their magic by affecting the production of hormone-like molecules called prostaglandins. Some kinds of prostaglandins are pro-inflammatory while others, like those derived from the Omega-3s in salmon are anti-inflammatory. The primary Omega-3 found in salmon, eicosapentaenoic acid (EPA), is the immediate precursor of the Series 3 prostaglandins, an anti-inflammatory type that prevents platelets from sticking together and improves blood flow. A four ounce serving of salmon contains 33.6% of the daily value for Omega-3 fatty acids.

One healthy result of fish consumption, especially when the fish consumed are rich in Omega-3 fats, is a lower risk of stroke. A recent study, which involved almost 80,000 nurses during a 15-year period, revealed that those women who ate fish 2-4 times per week had a 27% reduced risk of stroke compared to women who ate fish once a month. Those who ate fish five or more times per week reduced their risk of certain strokes 52%.

Heavyweight Healing Foods—CONTINUED

Salmon promotes cardiovascular health not only through its concentration of Omega-3 fats, but also because this fish is a very good source of the B-vitamins, niacin and Vitamin B12. Niacin, which is necessary for the chemical processing of fats in the body, has been repeatedly used clinically to successfully lower total blood cholesterol in individuals with elevated cholesterol levels. Vitamin B12 plays a critical role as a methyl donor. *Methylation* is a basic cellular process in which methyl groups are transferred from one molecule to another, resulting in the formation of a wide variety of very important active molecules. When levels of B12 are inadequate, the availability of methyl groups is also lessened. One result of the lack of methyl groups is that molecules that would normally be quickly changed into other types of molecules do not change and they accumulate. One such molecule, homocysteine, is so damaging to blood vessel walls that high levels are considered a significant risk factor for cardiovascular disease. Just four ounces of baked or broiled salmon provide 56.7% of the daily value for niacin and 54.2% of the daily value for Vitamin B12.

Description of Salmon

While salmon are born in fresh water, they spend a good portion of their lives in the sea, only to navigate hundreds of miles to return to their birthplace in order to spawn. It's no wonder that these smart and intuitive fish are considered a "brain food."

Salmon are usually classified either as Pacific (*Oncorhynchus* family) or Atlantic (*Salmo* family) salmon, according to the ocean in which they are found. There is just one species of Atlantic salmon, while there are five species of Pacific salmon including *chinook* (or king), *sockeye* (or red), *coho* (or silver), *pink* and *chum*. Norwegian salmon, a popular type of salmon often offered on restaurant menus, is actually Atlantic salmon that is farm-raised in Norway.

History of Salmon

People have been enjoying salmon as a food ever since this beautiful fish appeared in the Earth's waters—basically, since time immemorial. Much of the salmon available in today's market comes from the waters of Alaska, the Pacific Northwest, eastern Canada, Norway and Greenland.

Like other fish, in addition to being consumed fresh, preservation techniques such as smoking or salting were used to preserve the salmon. Smoked salmon is still considered traditional fare in the cuisines of Scandinavia and the Russian Federation.

How to Select Salmon

Salmon is sold in many different forms. Fresh salmon is available whole or in steak or fillet form. Salmon is also available frozen, canned, dried or smoked.

Always choose wild rather than farm raised salmon. Research published by the *Environmental Working Group* indicates that farmed salmon poses a cancer risk because it may be carrying high levels of carcinogenic chemicals called *polychlorinated biphenyls* (PCBs). PCBs have been banned in the U.S. for use in all but completely closed areas since 1979, but they persist in the environment and end up in animal fat. When farmed salmon from U.S. grocery stores was tested, the farmed salmon, which contains up to twice

Heavyweight Healing Foods—CONTINUED

the fat of wild salmon, was found to contain 16 times the PCBs found in wild salmon, 4 times the levels in beef, and 3.4 times the levels found in other seafood. Other studies done in Canada, Ireland and Britain have produced similar findings.

Safety of Salmon

Government inspection is not mandated for seafood, so choose your fish purveyor carefully. While some fish are not considered safe for pregnant or nursing mothers or young children to eat, eating wild pacific salmon does not pose a safety concern.

SEA VEGETABLES

Western cultures are only recently beginning to enjoy the taste and nutritional value of sea vegetables, often referred to as seaweed. They have been a staple of the Japanese diet for centuries. Many varieties of sea vegetables can be found in health food and specialty stores throughout the year and are also becoming much easier to find in your local supermarkets with their rise in popularity.

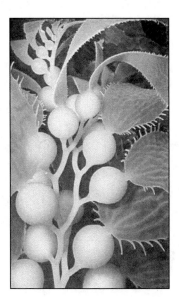

Sea vegetables can be found growing both in the marine salt waters as well as in fresh water lakes and seas. They commonly grow on coral reefs or in rocky landscapes, and can grow at great depths provided that sunlight can penetrate through the water to where they reside since, like plants, they need light for their survival. Sea vegetables are neither plants nor animals but classified in a group known as *algae*.

Health Benefits of Sea Vegetables

Why would anyone want to eat seaweed? Because sea vegetables offer the broadest range of minerals of any food, containing virtually all the minerals found in the ocean — the same minerals that are found in human blood. Sea vegetables are a very good source of the B-vitamin folate, and magnesium, and a good source of iron, calcium, and the B-vitamins riboflavin and pantothenic acid. In addition, seaweeds contain good amounts of lignans, plant compounds with cancer-protective properties.

Promote Healthy Thyroid Function with Sea Vegetables

Sea vegetables, especially kelp, are nature's richest sources of iodine, which as a component of the thyroid hormones thyroxine (T4) and triiodothyronine (T3), is essential to human life. The thyroid gland adds iodine to the amino acid tyrosine to create these hormones. Without sufficient iodine, your body cannot synthesize them. Because these thyroid hormones regulate metabolism in every cell of the body and play a role in virtually all physiological functions, an iodine deficiency can have a devastating impact on your health and well-being. A common sign of thyroid deficiency is an enlarged thyroid gland, commonly called a goiter. Goiters are estimated to affect 200 million people worldwide, and in all but 4% of these cases, the cause is iodine deficiency.

Heavyweight Healing Foods—CONTINUED

Description of Sea Vegetables

Sea vegetables, often called seaweed, are one of the Neptune's beautiful jewels, adorning the waters with life and providing us with a food that can enhance our diets, from both a culinary and nutritional perspective. Sea vegetables can be found growing both in the marine salt waters as well as in fresh water lakes and seas. They commonly grow on coral reefs or in rocky landscapes, and can grow at great depths provided that sunlight can penetrate through the water to where they reside since, like plants, they need light for their survival. Yet sea vegetables are neither plants nor animals they are actually known as algae.

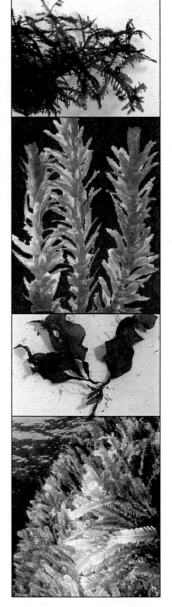

There are thousands of types of sea vegetables that are classified into categories by color, known either as brown, red or green sea vegetables. Each is unique, having a distinct shape, taste and texture. Although not all sea vegetables that exist are presently consumed, a wide range of sea vegetables are enjoyed as foods. The following are some of the most popular types:

- ▶ **Nori:** dark purple-black color that turns phosphorescent green when toasted, famous for its role in making sushi rolls.

- ▶ **Kelp:** light brown to dark green in color, oftentimes available in flake form.

- ▶ **Hijiki:** looks like small strands of black wiry pasta, has a strong flavor.

- ▶ **Kombu:** very dark in color and generally sold in strips or sheets, often used as a flavoring for soups.

- ▶ **Wakame:** similar to Kombu, most commonly used to make Japanese miso soup.

- ▶ **Arame:** this lacy, wiry sea vegetable is sweeter and milder in taste than many others.

- ▶ **Dulse:** soft, chewy texture and a reddish-brown color.

History of Sea Vegetables

The consumption of sea vegetables enjoys a long history throughout the world. Archaeological evidence suggests that Japanese cultures have been consuming sea vegetables for more than 10,000 years. In ancient Chinese cultures, sea vegetables were a noted delicacy, suitable especially for honored guests and royalty. Yet, sea vegetables were not just limited to being a featured part of Asian cuisines. In fact, most regions and countries located by waters, including Scotland, Ireland, Norway, Iceland, New Zealand, the Pacific Islands and coastal South American countries have been consuming sea vegetables since ancient times. Presently, Japan is the largest producer and exporter of sea vegetables. This may explain why many of these precious foods are often called by their Japanese names.

Heavyweight Healing Foods—CONTINUED

How to Select and Store Sea Vegetables

Look for sea vegetables that are sold in tightly sealed packages. Avoid those that have evidence of excessive moisture. Some types of sea vegetables are sold in different forms. For example, nori can be found in sheets, flakes, or powder. Choose the form of sea vegetables that will best meet your culinary needs.

Store sea vegetables in tightly sealed containers at room temperature where they can stay fresh for at least several months.

Safety of Sea Vegetables

Sea vegetables are not a commonly allergenic food, are not included in the list of 20 foods that most frequently contain pesticide residues, and are also not known to contain *goitrogens, oxalates,* or *purines.*

TEMPEH

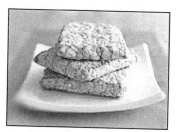

Although not a common item in most households in the U.S., the distinctively nutty taste and nougat-like texture of tempeh is increasing in popularity. It easily absorbs the flavors of the other foods with which it is cooked making it adaptable to many types of dishes. Tempeh can be found in health food stores and specialty markets throughout the year.

Tempeh has been a staple in Indonesia for over 2000 years. It is typically made by cooking and dehulling soybeans, inoculating them with a culturing agent (like *Rhizopus oligosporus*), and then incubating the innoculated product overnight until it forms a solid cake. It is a highly nutritious fermented food traditionally made from soybeans and its high protein content makes it a wonderful substitute for meat.

Health Benefits of Tempeh

The soybean is the most widely grown and utilized legume in the world, with the U.S. being responsible for more than 50% of the world's production of this important food. Soy is one the most widely researched, health-promoting foods around. A complete review of all the benefits soy foods offer could easily fill a large book. Soy's key benefits are related to its excellent protein content, its high levels of essential fatty acids, numerous vitamins and minerals, its isoflavones, and its fiber. Tempeh provides not only the protein found in soybeans but many other health benefits as well.

A Healthy Transition Through Menopause

One of the more popular uses of soy foods lately has been in the treatment of menopausal symptoms. Soybeans contain active compounds called isoflavones that act like very weak estrogens in the body. These phytoestrogens bind to estrogen receptors and may provide enough stimulation to help eliminate some of the uncomfortable symptoms that occur when natural estrogen levels decline. Studies have shown that women who consume soy foods report a significant reduction in the amount of hot flashes that they experience. There is also some evidence that soy foods may even be able to help reduce the bone loss that typically occurs after menopause. And as women's risk for heart disease significantly increases at menopause, soy foods' numerous beneficial cardiovascular effects make tempeh a particularly excellent choice for frequent consumption as menopause approaches.

Eating For Health™ Your Guide to Vitality & Optimal Health

Heavyweight Healing Foods—CONTINUED

History of Tempeh

Shortly after colonizing Indonesia, the Dutch introduced tempeh and other native foodstuffs into Europe. It was not until the 20th century that this Southeast Asian delight was introduced into the United States. Tempeh is now gaining increased popularity in this country as people look for ways to increase their intake of soybeans, and they discover tempeh's versatility and delicious taste.

How to Select and Store Tempeh

For many years it was only possible to find tempeh in natural foods and Asian stores. Yet, with the growing demand for soy foods, tempeh is now becoming more and more available in supermarkets throughout the country. Depending upon the store, tempeh may either be kept in the refrigerated or freezer section. In addition to plain soy tempeh, often varieties that include grains or vegetables are available.

Look for tempeh that is covered with a thin whitish bloom. While it may have a few black or grayish spots, it should have no evidence of pink, yellow or blue coloration as this indicates that it has become overly fermented.

Refrigerated tempeh can keep in the refrigerator for up to ten days. If you do not consume the whole package of tempeh at one time, wrap it well and place it back in the refrigerator. Tempeh will keep fresh for several months in the freezer.

Safety of Tempeh

As a soy-based food, tempeh contains *goitrogens*, naturally occurring substances in certain foods that can interfere with the functioning of the thyroid gland. Individuals with already existing and untreated thyroid problems may want to limit consumption of tempeh for this reason. Cooking may help to inactivate the goitrogenic compounds found in tempeh.

Tempeh is among a small number of foods that contain any measurable amount of *oxalates*, naturally occurring substances found in plants, animals, and human beings. When oxalates become too concentrated in body fluids, they can crystallize and cause health problems. For this reason, individuals with already existing and untreated kidney or gallbladder problems may want to limit consumption of tempeh.

Oxalates may also interfere with absorption of calcium from the body. For this reason, individuals trying to increase their calcium stores may want to avoid consuming tempeh at the same time as calcium-rich foods, or if taking calcium supplements, may want to consume tempeh 2-3 hours before or after taking their supplements.

Individuals who suspect food allergy to be an underlying factor in their health problems may want to avoid commonly allergenic foods. Soybeans and products like tempeh that are made from them are among the foods most commonly associated with allergic reactions.

Adapted from the *World's Healthiest Foods* (www.whfoods.com). Thanks to The George Mateljan Foundation for a their outstanding research and public service in this area. References at www.whfoods.com

Top Twelve Power Foods

by Edward Bauman, M.Ed., Ph.D.

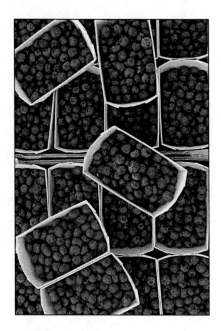

Avocado: Reduces risk of heart attack. Aids in blood and tissue regeneration. High in protein, phosphorus, magnesium, calcium, and manganese. Stabilizes blood sugar and excellent for heart disorders.

Beets: Richer than spinach in iron and other minerals. One of the best foods to relieve constipation. Good for obesity. Aid digestion, as well as lymphatic, gall bladder, and liver function. Also aid anemia by helping to build red blood cells.

Blueberry: Unusual type of antibiotic action, blocking attachment of bacteria that cause urinary tract infections. Also has anti-viral activity. Contains silicon, which helps rejuvenate the pancreas. Good for diabetic conditions.

Cabbage (including broccoli and bok choy): Contains numerous anti-cancer and antioxidant compounds. Helps block breast cancer and suppress growth of polyps, a prelude to colon cancer. Eating cabbage more than once a week cut men's colon cancer odds 66%, and as little as two daily tablespoons of cooked cabbage protected against stomach cancer (Murray and Pizzorno, 2005). Contains anti-ulcer compounds; cabbage juice helps heal ulcers in humans. Kills bacteria and viruses. Stimulates the immune system. A good blood purifier and vitalizing agent.

Carrot: High in beta carotene, a powerful anti-cancer, artery-protecting, immune-boosting, infection-fighting antioxidant with wide protective powers. A carrot a day slashed stroke rates in women by 68%. The beta-carotene in one medium carrot cuts lung cancer risk in half, even among formerly heavy smokers (Murray and Pizzorno, 2005). Improves the eyesight. Beta carotene, as found in carrots, substantially reduces odds of degenerative eye diseases such as cataracts and macular degeneration. The high soluble fiber in carrots promotes regularity. Cooking can make it easier for the body to absorb carrot's beta-carotene. Builds healthy skin and tissue. Good for heart disease. Reduces the risk of cancer.

Celery: A traditional remedy for high blood pressure. Eat two to four stalks a day. Also has a mild diuretic effect. Contains eight different families of anti-cancer compounds that detoxify carcinogens. Aids digestion, as well as kidney and liver function. Good for blood sugar regulation. Reduces water retention. Helps regulate the nervous system.

Cranberry: An excellent curative and preventative therapy for the entire breathing apparatus. Contain a natural vasodilator, which opens the bronchial tubes. Long used for its powers against bacterial infections and viruses of the bladder, kidneys, and urinary tract.

Top Twelve Power Foods—CONTINUED

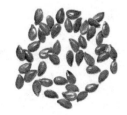

Flax seed: Used primarily for constipation. Helps with gastritis, colitis, or other inflammations of the digestive tract. Lowers blood fat levels often associated with heart attacks and strokes. Its soluble fibers reduce harmful blood cholesterol levels. Rich source of lignans, a documented anti-cancer agent that prevents colon and breast cancer. Improves moods, diminishes allergies, and produces healthier skin.

Fish and fish oil: An ounce a day cut risk of heart attacks by 50% (Murray and Pizzorno, 2005). Omega-3 fatty acids in fish can relieve symptoms of rheumatoid arthritis, osteoarthritis, asthma, psoriasis, and high blood pressure. A known anti-inflammatory agent and anti-coagulant. Raises good HDL cholesterol. Lowers triglycerides. Guards against glucose intolerance and Type II diabetes. Some fish are high in antioxidants, such as selenium and coenzyme Q-10. Exhibits anti-cancer activity, especially blocking development of colon cancer and spread of breast cancer. Fish highest in Omega-3 fatty acids include sardines, mackerel, herring, salmon, and tuna.

Garlic: Broad-spectrum antibiotic that combats bacteria, intestinal parasites, and viruses. Lowers blood pressure and blood cholesterol, discourages dangerous blood clotting. Two or three cloves a day cut the odds of subsequent heart attacks in half in heart patients. Contains multiple anti-cancer compounds and antioxidants, topping the National Cancer Institute's list of a potential cancer-preventing food. Lessens risk of stomach cancer in particular. A good cold medication, acting as a decongestant, expectorant, and anti-inflammatory agent. Boosts immune response.

Mushroom (maitake and shiitake): Enhances immune function. Used as a longevity tonic, heart medicine, and cancer remedy in Asia. Current research shows that mushrooms, such as maitake, help prevent and/or treat cancer, viral diseases, high cholesterol, and high blood pressure. Eaten daily, maitake or shiitake, fresh (three ounces) or dried (one-third ounce), cut cholesterol by 7% and 12%, respectively (Murray and Pizzorno, 2005). Used to treat leukemia in China and breast cancer in Japan.

Seaweed: One of the best foods to nourish the thyroid; its iodine content helps prevent goiter. Rich in important minerals, so helpful against many degenerative diseases. Benefits include reducing blood cholesterol and helping disorders of the genito-urinary and reproductive systems. Kelp has anti-bacterial and anti-viral activity. Most types of seaweed have anti-cancer activity. Studies show that some seaweeds (including arame, hiziki, and kombu) can help remove radioactive elements from the body (Murray and Pizzorno, 2005). Long acclaimed as beauty aids as they help maintain beautiful skin and lustrous hair.

Top Twelve Power Foods—CONTINUED

Health-Enhancing Herbs and Spices

Fenugreek seed: A spice common in the Middle East and available in many U.S. food markets. Has anti-diabetic powers, helping to control surges of blood sugar and insulin. Has anti-cancer properties and tends to lower blood pressure. Helps prevent intestinal gas.

Ginger: Classic tonic for the digestive tract. Stimulates digestion and keeps the intestinal muscles toned. Acts as an anti-inflammatory agent, so can relieve symptoms of arthritis. Supports a healthy cardiovascular system.

Parsley: Anti-cancer because of high levels of antioxidants. Good for purifying the blood and stimulating the bowel. Rich in iron, copper, and manganese. Makes an excellent tea and helps to release retained water. Builds the blood and stimulates brain activity.

Turmeric: A marvelous medicinal spice. Its main active ingredient is curcumin, which gives turmeric its intense cadmium yellow color. Curcumin is an anti-inflammatory agent on a par with cortisone and can reduce symptoms of rheumatoid arthritis. Helps to lower cholesterol. Protects the liver from toxins, boosts stomach defenses against acid, lowers blood sugar in diabetics, and acts as a powerful anti-cancer agent.

Remember to buy organic foods whenever possible!

Murray, Michael T.; Pizzorno, Joseph; and Pizzorno, Lara (2005). *The Encyclopedia of Healing Foods*. New York: Atria Books (a division of Simon & Schuster).

Booster Foods

SPIRULINA

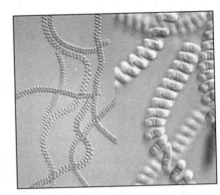

Origin of Spirulina

Spirulina is relatively new to North Americans. However, Aztecs ate it as a staple food, mixed with maize. Natives of the sahara dry it with grains, vegetables, and seasonings to form a meal in itself.[1]

Ancient cultures were aware of spirulina's exceptional life-generating energy and held its remarkable energizing and rejuvenating properties in high esteem The Aztecs harvested this "superfood" into what they called "blue mud" from Lake Texcoco and dried it into loaves. The Aztecs considered it a "Sacred Power Plant." Priests and warriors sustained themselves (at times solely) on dried spirulina wafers.[2]

Nutritional Value of Spirulina

Spirulina produces all its nutrients by harvesting sunlight. It gathers and transforms sunlight into green and blue pigments that make it a blue green algae. The blue is an amino acid group found only in Spirulina called *phycocyanin*, which accounts for its high concentration of vegetarian protein. The green in Spirulina is *chlorophyll*, one of the best natural detoxifiers known. Spirulina is a balanced natural whole food. It's minerals and vitamins are naturally bio-chelated, meaning they are wrapped in amino-acids for excellent assimilation by the body. It contains over 100 synergistic nutrients and is nature's richest and most complete source of total organic nutrition. Spirulina is a completely natural, and therefore superior, approach to nutrition.

Health Benefits of Spirulina

Scientific studies world-wide have demonstrated the incredible anti-cancer properties of Spirulina.

Spirulina is a rich source *Gamma Linolenic Acid* (GLA), which is its "miracle" ingredient. GLA is an essential fatty acid that has been shown very helpful in the relief of arthritis and also helps lower high blood pressure and blood cholesterol.

It eases other conditions such as premenstrual pain, eczema and other skin conditions. It is a powerful Immune System Builder and extremely detoxifying.[3]

Spirulina has been scientifically demonstrated to increase the reproduction of lacto-bacilli, the bacteria that digests our food. Therefore it improves the gastrointestinal and digestive health.

Nutrition Facts

SPIRULINA / 1 CUP DRIED	
Calories	44
Protein (g)	9
Carbohydrate (g)	4
Dietary Fiber (g)	1
Total Fat (g)	1.2
Potassium (mg)	204
Sodium (mg)	157
Thiamin (mg)	.36
Riboflavin (mg)	.55
Niacin (mg)	1.9
Folate (mcg)	14.1
Iron (mg)	4.3
Magnesium (mg)	29.3

SOURCE: Margen[11]

Booster Foods—CONTINUED

NUTRITIONAL YEAST

Origin of Nutritional Yeast

Yeast belongs to the same family as edible mushrooms and the beneficial organisms used for medical and veterinary use. It may be considered man's oldest industrial micro-organism. With the invention of the microscope, it became possible to isolate yeast in pure culture form. The pioneering scientific work of Louis Pasteur in the late 1860s has resulted in the ability today to commercially produce baker's yeast, wine yeast, and nutritional yeast.

Nutritional Yeast *(Saccharomyces cerevisiae)* is a primary grown nutritional yeast grown specifically for nutritional benefits.

Active Dry Yeast is made from cream yeast. It is a raising agent used in baked goods.

Brewers Yeast, is a bitter by-product of the brewing industry that has a high nutritional profile, but typically not as high as nutritional yeast which is grown for maximized nutritional benefits.

Health Benefits of Nutritional Yeast

Sprinkling nutritional yeast in their food is a good way to repel fleas from dogs and cats. Besides being very healthy for the dog/cat, the smell they secrete will be very nasty to flees.

Yeast is well known for its B-complex vitamins, which are essential to the wellness of body, mind, and spirit. *Thiamin* (B1) deficiency can lead to hand and foot numbness as well as damage to the central nervous system. Vegetarians, diabetics, and women taking birth control pills are highly susceptible to *Riboflavin* (B2) deficiency.

Niacin (B3) and *Pyridoxine* (B6) are needed for the production of antibodies and red blood cells, and promotes a normal functioning nervous and musculoskeletal system.

Cyanocobalamin (B12) helps prevent nerve damage and anemia, aids in cell and blood formation, proper digestion, fertility and growth. This vitamin is also helpful during pregnancy and lactation. Vegetarians and immune compromised individuals are the most at risk of Vitamin B12 deficiency.

Nutrition Facts

NUTRITIONAL YEAST/ 2 TBSP. /16G.	
Calories	60
Protein (g)	8.34
Carbohydrate (g)	7.2
Dietary Fiber (g)	3.9
Total Fat (g)	0.83
Potassium (mg)	320
Sodium (mg)	5.12
Calcium (mg)	11.2
Iron (mg)	0.77
Thiamin (B1) (mg)	9.6
Riboflavin (B2) (mg)	9.6
Niacin (mg)	56
Vitamin B6 (mg)	9.6
Folic Acid (mcg)	240
Vitamin B12 (mcg)	8
Biotin (mcg)	20.8
Pantothenic Acid (mg)	1.04
Phosphorus (mg)	174.4
Magnesium (mg)	20.8
Zinc (mg)	3.2
Selenium (mcg)	22.4
Copper (mg)	0.128
Manganese (mg)	0.094
Chromium (mg)	< 0.5
Molybdenum (mcg)	6.4

SOURCE: Margen[11]

Booster Foods—CONTINUED

HEALING HERBS

GINGER

Origin of Ginger

No one really knows the exact origins of ginger. It was probably first discovered in the tropics of Southeast Asia.[4] Now this plant is grown in the East Indies, Mexico, Jamaica, and Africa and is most prized for its rhizome (an underground stem).

The Spanish explores brought ginger from the East Indies into Spain in the 16th century. It was a delicacy and sold in various parts of Europe. For thousands of years, trade in spices like ginger became the measure of an empire's wealth and power. The Spanish people, who were particularly aggressive explorers and colonialists, were one of the key nations responsible for taking ginger around the globe and encouraging its cultivation in the New World.[4]

Ginger Folklore

The *Traditional Chinese Medicine* and *Ayurvedic Indian Systems* clearly viewed ginger as a healing gift from God. The most ancient Chinese pharmacopoeias, claimed that long term usage of fresh ginger would put a person in contact with the spiritual effulgences. In ancient India, it was the universal medicine. Centuries later, the sacred writings of the Koran declared ginger a beverage of the holiest heavenly spirits.[4] Ginger was used in medieval European cookery as a preservative, and it was also used to mask the meat when it was old or bad.

Health Benefits of Ginger[4]

Ginger is capable of invigorating and balancing a wide range of body systems, from the circulatory and respiratory systems to the reproductive organs.

Ginger has the ability to:

▶ Normalize blood sugar and cholesterol

▶ Stimulates and tones the circulatory, respiratory, immune and reproductive systems

▶ Reduce levels of *eicosanoids,* hence lessening in inflammation and fever

▶ Relief from osteoarthritis and rheumatoid arthritis

▶ Enhance motility

▶ Stimulate the hormonal level of the body

Energetics

Ginger is warming, pungent, and spicy.[4]

Nutrition Facts

GINGER / 2 TABLESPOONS SLICED	
Calories	8
Protein (g)	>1
Carbohydrate (g)	2
Dietary Fiber (g)	0.2
Total Fat (g)	0.1
Potassium (mg)	50
Sodium (mg)	2

SOURCE: Margen[11]

Booster Foods—CONTINUED

OREGANO

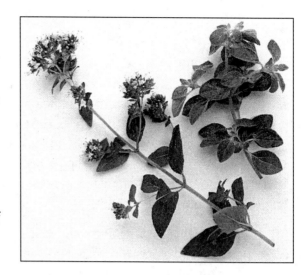

Origin of Oregano

Oregano is considered the quintessential Italian Herb. It is a relative of mint and is commonly used in Mediterranean and Mexican cooking. In Britain the same plant is known as wild marjoram. It was taken to America by the early settlers, where its name was changed in the 1940s.[5]

Oregano Folklore

The Greeks termed the spice *origanos,* meaning "delight of the mountains." The hillsides are covered with oregano and scents the summer air in Greece. The sweet, spicy scent of Oregano was reputedly created by the Goddess Aphrodite as a symbol of happiness. Bridal couples were crowned with garlands of oregano, and the plants were placed on the tombs to give peace to departed spirits.[6]

Nutritional Value of Oregano

The compound in Oregano, *rosmarinic acid,* has antibacterial, anti-inflammatory, antioxidant and antiviral properties. Of all the plants in the mint family, Oregano is the richest in antioxidants.

Health Benefits of Oregano

Oregano prevents the cell damage caused by free-radicals. Free-radical reactions are most likely involved in inflammation, degenerative arthritis and the aging process in general. Evidence is growing that antioxidants may help relieve osteoarthritis and rheumatism. Oregano is helpful in combating diarrhea, intestinal gas and digestive problems.[6] Oregano is loaded with antiseptic compounds. Therefore it is useful in treating sinusitus[6] and all respiratory problems, coughs, bronchitis, and even asthma.[5]

Oregano contains:

▶ Four anti-asthmatic compounds
▶ Six compounds that are expectorants
▶ Seven that lower blood pressure
▶ Nineteen antibacterial compounds

Nutrition Facts

GROUND OREGANO / 1 TABLESPOON	
Calories	14
Protein (g)	0
Carbohydrate (g)	3
Dietary Fiber (g)	2
Total Fat (g)	.5
Potassium (mg)	
Sodium (mg)	1

SOURCE: Margen[11]

Uses for Oregano

Used in omeletts, tomato dishes, salads, sauces, stews and vegetables.

Booster Foods—CONTINUED

ROSEMARY

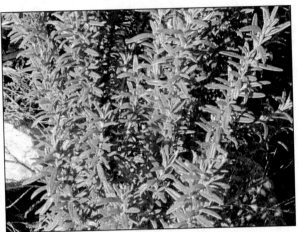

Origin of Rosemary

Rosemary belongs to the mint family. Its native habitat is the area around the Mediterranean Sea and Portugal. It is now cultivated in many countries. Rosemary can grow to be 6 feet tall and grows out to look like bushes. The leaves are long and skinny like pine needles. Rosemary flowers, which are violet in color, bloom briefly in spring on young shoots.

Commercially cultivated and dried rosemary leaves come from Spain, France, Morocco, and Tunisia. The leaves have essential oils, which contain tannin and resin.[7]

Rosemary Folklore

The origin of this herbs name is woven into folklore. It is said that the Virgin Mary had draped her cloak over this bush and placed a white flower on top of her cloak. In the morning the flower turned blue and thereafter the plant was called "Rose of Mary."

Rosemary was introduced to the Alps in the middle ages and became part of many folk customs. People burned rosemary and inhaled the smoke to ward off sickness. Broken sprigs of rosemary were used for baptisms, funerals and marriages.[7] In Europe, wedding parties burned Rosemary as incense.

Health Benefits of Rosemary

Rosemary is anti-inflammatory and it stimulates the gall bladder and increases the flow of bile, aiding fat digestion. It also aids good circulation and strengthens weak blood vessels.

The *rosamaricene* acts as a mild painkiller. Rosemary tea is an excellent natural remedy for headaches. It is an effective remedy for depression and despondency. It is used in many herbal shampoos.[5]

Uses for Rosemary

The fragrant leaves are used to flavor stews, tomato sauces, potatoes, soups, vegetables, salmon, tuna and lamb dishes. It is also mixed with food that spoils easily.[5]

Nutrition Facts

DRIED ROSEMARY / 1 TABLESPOON	
Calories	11
Protein (g)	0
Carbohydrate (g)	2
Dietary Fiber (g)	1
Total Fat (g)	0.5
Potassium (mg)	0
Sodium (mg)	2

SOURCE: Margen[11]

Booster Foods—CONTINUED

PARSLEY

Origins of Parsley

Parsley was cultivated as early as the third century B.C. The Romans used Parsley as a garnish and flavoring. It spread to the Americas in the 17th century, where it now grows plentifully. Some say it originated in the Mediterranean — possibly Sardinia.

Parsley Folklore

The Romans put parsley on their tables and around their necks in the belief the leaves would absorb fumes. Medieval Europeans believed that one could kill an enemy by plucking a sprig while speaking the person's name.[9]

Health Benefits of Parsley

Parsley is traditionally used as a diuretic and anti-inflammatory and is also a strong antioxidant. It aids the elimination of uric acid, therefore it is useful in treating rheumatism and gout.[5]

Uses for Parsley

Parsley's appealing flavor makes it a component of both the traditional fines herbes and bouquet garni flavorings of French cooking. It is a favorite flavoring for egg dishes, vegetable dishes, pastas and soups and it is a traditional garnish. The herb is very nutritious with high iron and vitamin levels.[10]

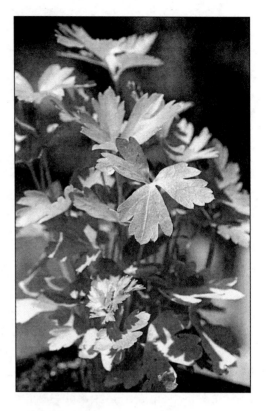

Nutrition Facts

PARSLEY / 1/4 CUP CHOPPED RAW	
Calories	
Protein (g)	
Carbohydrate (g)	
Dietary Fiber (g)	
Total Fat (g)	
Potassium (mg)	83
Sodium (mg)	
Beta carotene	0.5
Vitamin C	20
Folate (mcg)	23
Iron (mg)	0.9

SOURCE: Margen[11]

Booster Foods—CONTINUED

HEALING FRUITS

APPLES

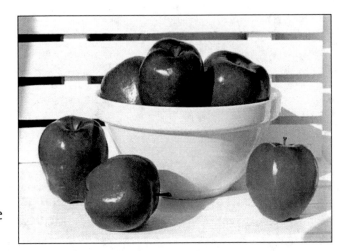

Origin of Apples

Fossil remains have shown that apples were gathered and stored 5,000 years ago, and it is likely that they were already being cultivated in Neolithic times. The Egyptians grew apples, and invading Roman legions introduced them to Britain. The early colonists brought apples to America from their home country, establishing orchards in Massachusetts and Virginia; these became the foundation for most of the apples grown in the United States today.

Apple Folklore

"An apple a day keeps the doctor away." No fruit, and possibly no food, plays a more prominent role in religion, myth, folklore, and literature than does the apple. Apples symbolize knowledge and simultaneous treachery. Apples are beloved and cherished — and poisoned. We eat an apple and fall from grace. An apple falls from a tree as a physicist dozes, and a new revolution awakens in the world of science.

Health Benefits of Apples

▶ Apples contain soluble fiber — *pectin,* a fiber that keeps the bowels functioning properly and lowers cholesterol.[5]

▶ Apples protect against environmental pollutants.

▶ Apples contain *malic* and *tartaric* acids, which aid digestion and are especially helpful in dealing with rich, fatty foods.

▶ Apples' Vitamin C helps to boost the body's own immune defenses[5]

▶ Apples heal intestinal infections, inflammation of the colon, diarrhea, arthritis, herpes and viruses

▶ Apples protect against danger from x-rays and radiation therapy[8]

▶ Apples are a major dietary source of an antioxidant phytochemical called quercetin, which may have cancer protection, allergy symptom relief, and anti-clotting effects.[11]

Nutrition Facts

APPLE / 1 LARGE WITH PEEL	
Calories	125
Protein (g)	>1
Carbohydrate (g)	32
Dietary Fiber (g)	5.7
Total Fat (g)	0.8
Potassium (mg)	243
Vitamin C (mg)	12

SOURCE: Margen[11]

Booster Foods—CONTINUED

APRICOTS

Origin of Apricots

These golden, fragrant, delicate fruits originated in China about 4,000 years ago and were transplanted throughout Asia and Europe. The Romans introduced apricots to Europe in 70-60 B.C. through Greece and Italy. In the late 1700s, the Spanish introduced apricots to California, where they were planted in the gardens of Spanish mission. Today, California supplies.about 95% of the apricots grown in the United States.[11]

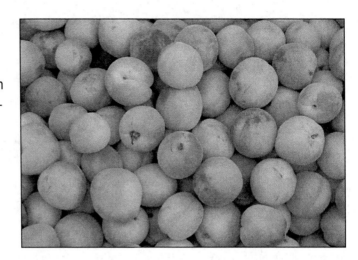

Apricot Folklore

The apricot was used to symbolize female genitalia just like the peach and other stone fruits. In medieval France, the word *abricot* was slang for vulva.

Health Benefits of Apricots

Apricots contain large amounts of beta-carotene, which the body converts to Vitamin A.[5] Apricots help prevent cancer and also improve:

- ▶ Constipation and all bowel disorders
- ▶ Muscle and nerve tissue
- ▶ Skin[8]

Nutrition Facts

FRESH APRICOTS / 3	
Calories	50
Protein (g)	2
Carbohydrate (g)	12
Dietary Fiber (g)	2.5
Total Fat (g)	0.4
Potassium (mg)	1.6
Vitamin C (mg)	11

SOURCE: Margen[11]

Booster Foods—CONTINUED

BLUEBERRIES

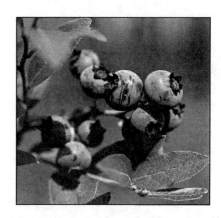

Origin of Blueberries

This shrub is native to both Europe and North America.[5] Blueberries have probably been collected by native people for thousands of years in North America, and later by European settlers, but were domesticated only in the twentieth century. Prior to 1900, selection of bushes from the wild was known to have occurred. Plantsmen and plant breeders, notably Frederick Coville, selected and bred large-fruited cultivars after the turn of the century, which formed the foundation of the modern industry.

Health Benefits of Blueberries

Blueberries contain the antibacterial anthocyanosides, which have a tonic effect on blood vessels and make them a useful aid in the treatment of varicose veins. In addition, they help in the treatment of cystitis and other urinary infections.[5] Blueberries are rich in antioxidants, which are potential cancer-fighters.[11] Flavonoid phytochemicals may make blood platelets less likely to stick together and from the type of clots that can cause heart attacks.[11] Blueberries are good for:

- ▶ Food poisoning and diarrhea.[5]
- ▶ Rejuvenating the pancreas[8]
- ▶ Blue pigment may be a powerful liver protector[8]
- ▶ Tinnitus[8]

Nutrition Facts

BLUEBERRIES ˜/ 1 CUP	
Calories	81
Protein (g)	1
Carbohydrate (g)	21
Dietary Fiber (g)	3.9
Total Fat (g)	0.6
Potassium (mg)	129
Vitamin C (mg)	19
Vitamin E	2.7

SOURCE: Margen[11]

REFERENCES
1. Roehl, Evelyn. *Whole Food Facts.* Healing Arts Press, VT. 1996.
2. www.dietblends.com/information/ingredients.cfm
3. www.spirulina.com
4. Schulick, Paul. *Ginger.* Herbal Free Press Ltd. VT. 1996
5. Van Straten, Michael. *Healing Foods.* Welcome Rain, NY. 1997
6. www.survival.com.mx/health/oregano/moreinfo.html
7. http://vtvt.essortment.com/whatisrosemary_rqlg.htm
8. Balch, Phyllis and James. C.N.C and M.D. *Prescription for Dietary Wellness.* Avery Publishing Group. N.Y. 1998.
9. www.culinarycafe.com/Spices_Herbs/Parsley.html
10. www.global-garden.com.au/gardenherbs4.htm)
11. Margen, Sheldon M.D. *Wellness Foods A to Z.* Rebus, Inc. NY. 2002
12. www.uga.edu/fruit/bluberi

BIBLIOGRAPHY
Murray, Michael N.D. *The Healing Power of Foods.* Prima Publishing, Rocklin, CA. 1993.
Pitchford, Paul. *Healing With Whole Foods.* North Atlantic Books, Berkeley, CA. 1993.
The NutriBase Nutrition Facts Desk Reference. Second Edition. NY. Avery. 2002.

Medicinal Value of Whole Foods

Be sure to buy organic produce whenever possible!

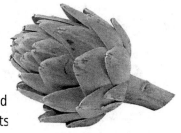

Alfalfa: Excellent for its alkalinizing effect. It is the richest source of chlorophyll. It is good for arthritis, promotes hair growth and is also good for congestion and respiratory disorders. It is high in nutrients because its roots travel down as deep as 250 feet into the clean deep earth.

Apple: Apples are good for elimination. They help to lower cholesterol and the risk of cancer. Apples are high in calcium and contain 50% more Vitamin C than oranges. Vitamin C helps to ward of colds and other infections. The apple helps to maintain nerve health.

Artichoke: High in fiber, calcium and iron. Excellent for the digestive tract, as well as heart, blood pressure, and blood sugar levels. They are good to eat for reduction of weight.

Asparagus: Many of the elements that build the liver, kidneys, skin, ligaments, and bones are found in green asparagus. It is a good vegetable for an elimination diet. Builds red blood cells and protects against cancer.

Avocado: Reduces the risk of heart attack and stabilizes blood sugars. Aids in blood and tissue regeneration. Avocados are high in protein, phosphorus, magnesium, calcium and manganese.

Banana: Soothes the stomach and strengthens the lining against acid and ulcers. Has antibiotic activity. Bananas feed the natural acidophilus bacteria of the bowel. Their high potassium content benefits the muscular system.

Beets: Richer than spinach in iron and other minerals. Beets are one of the best foods to relieve constipation. Good for obesity. Beets aid lymphatic, gall bladder and liver function. Also aids digestion, anemia and helps to build red blood cells.

Blueberry: Acts as an unusual type of antibiotic by blocking attachment of bacteria that cause urinary tract infections. Also has anti-viral activity. Contains silicon, which helps support the pancreas. They are good for diabetic conditions.

Broccoli: A unique package of versatile disease-fighters. Abundant in antioxidants, including quercetin, glutathione, beta carotene, Vitamin C and lutein. Extremely high in cancer fighting activity, particularly against lung, colon and breast cancers. Like other cruciferous vegetables, it speeds up removal of estrogen from the body, helping suppress breast cancer. Rich in cholesterol-reducing fiber. A super source of chromium that helps regulate insulin and blood sugar. Most protective when eaten raw or lightly cooked.

Cabbage (including bok choy): Contains numerous anti-cancer and antioxidant compounds. Helps block breast cancer and suppresses growth of polyps, a prelude to colon cancer. Eating cabbage more than once a week cuts men's colon cancer odds by 66%. As little as two daily tablespoons of cooked cabbage protects against stomach cancer. Contains anti-ulcer compounds and cabbage juice helps heal ulcers. Kills bacteria and viruses and stimulates the immune system. It is a good blood purifier and a vitalizing agent.

Medicinal Value of Whole Foods—CONTINUED

Carrot: High in *beta carotene*, a powerful anticancer, artery-protecting, immune-boosting, infection-fighting, antioxidant with wide protective powers. A carrot a day slashed stroke rates in women by 68%. The beta carotene in one medium carrot cuts lung cancer risk in half, even among formerly heavy smokers. Improves the eyesight and substantially reduces odds of degenerative eye diseases such as cataracts and macular degeneration. The high soluble fiber in carrots promotes regularity. Cooking can make it easier for the body to absorb carrot's beta carotene. Builds healthy skin and tissue, good for heart disease, and reduces the risk of cancer.

Cauliflower: Cruciferous family member that contains many of the same cancer-fighting, hormone-regulating compounds as its cousins, broccoli and cabbage. Eat raw, or lightly cooked. Reduces risk of cancer, particularly of the colon, rectum and stomach. Excellent for diabetes. Rich in Vitamin C, potassium and fiber.

Celery: A traditional remedy for high blood pressure. Eat two to four stalks a day. Also has a mild diuretic effect. Contains eight different families of anti-cancer compounds that detoxify carcinogens. Aids digestion, kidney and liver function, and helps regulate the nervous system. Also good for blood sugar regulation.

Chili pepper: Helps dissolve blood clots, opens up sinuses and air passages. Breaks up mucus in the lungs, and acts as an expectorant or decongestant. Helps prevent bronchitis, emphysema and stomach ulcers. Antibacterial, antioxidant activity. Putting hot chili sauce on food also speeds up metabolism, burning off calories.

Collard greens: Full of anti-cancer, antioxidant compounds, including lutein, Vitamin C and beta carotene. Like other green leafy vegetables, associated with low rates of all cancers.

Cranberry: An excellent preventive therapy for the entire breathing apparatus. Contains a natural vasodilator which opens up the bronchial tubes. Long used for its powers against bacterial infections and viruses of the bladder, kidneys and urinary tract.

Cucumbers: Should be eaten freely by people who live on the desert or in other hot climates — the most cooling food. Indicated for fevers, constipation, skin eruptions, high blood pressure, rheumatism, obesity, acidosis, and is a mild diuretic. A wonderful digestive aid and has a purifying effect on the bowel.

Dandelion greens: Dandelion greens are a wonderful liver cleanser and are valuable in helping the flow of the bile. Dandelion tea is an excellent drink for helping the liver and gall bladder. The greens stimulate the glands and help to relieve many toxic conditions of the skin.

Fenugreek seed: A spice common in the Middle East and available in many U.S. food markets. Has anti-diabetic powers, and helps control surges of blood sugar and insulin. Anti-cancer, tends to lower blood pressure. Helps prevent intestinal gas.

Medicinal Value of Whole Foods—CONTINUED

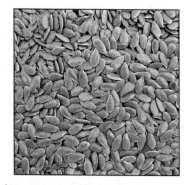

Flax seeds: Used primarily for constipation. Helps with gastritis, colitis or other inflammations of the digestive tract. Lowers blood fat levels often associated with heart attacks and strokes. Reduces harmful blood cholesterol levels with its soluble fibers. Prevents colon and breast cancer through its rich source of lignins, a documented anti-cancer agent. Improves moods, diminishes allergies and produces healthier skin.

Figs: Excellent natural laxative for sluggish bowels. A high source of dietary fiber that helps eliminate toxic wastes and mucus in the colon. One of the highest sources of calcium in the plant world. Gives nourishment and energy to the body.

Fish (wild and cold water): An ounce a day has been shown to cut risk of heart attacks by 50%. The Omega-3 oil in fish can relieve symptoms of rheumatoid arthritis, osteoarthritis, asthma, psoriasis, and high blood pressure. A known anti-inflammatory agent and anti-coagulant. Raises good type HDL cholesterol and lowers triglycerides. Guards against glucose intolerance and Type II diabetes. Some fish are high in antioxidants, such as selenium and Coenzyme Q-10. Exhibits anti-cancer activity especially in blocking development of colon cancer and spread of breast cancer. Fish highest in Omega-3 fatty acids include sardines, mackerel, herring, salmon, and tuna.

Garlic: Broad-spectrum antibiotic that combats bacteria, intestinal parasites and viruses. Lowers blood pressure and blood cholesterol, discourages dangerous blood clotting. Two or three cloves a day cut the odds of subsequent heart attacks by 50% in heart patients. Contains multiple anti-cancer compounds, antioxidants, and tops the *National Cancer Institute's* list as a potential cancer-preventive food. Lessens chances of stomach cancer in particular. A good cold medication, it acts as a decongestant, expectorant, and anti-inflammatory agent. Boosts immune responses.

Ginger: Ginger is a classic tonic for the digestive tract. It stimulates digestion and keeps the intestinal muscles toned. It acts as an anti-inflammatory agent and is useful with symptoms of arthritis. It also supports a healthy cardiovascular system.

Grapefruit: Has anticancer activity, and is particularly protective against stomach and pancreatic cancer. The juice is antiviral and high in various antioxidants, and is especially high in Vitamin C.

Grapes: Dark grapes are high in iron, which makes them a good blood builder. Grapes are wonderful for promoting action of the bowel, cleansing the liver, and aiding kidney function. They are soothing for the nervous system. A one day a week grape fast during the grape season is good for elimination.

Green beans: Helps with rheumatism. Increases urinary output. Energizes. Green beans have been found to promote the normal function of the liver and pancreas.

Kale: Rich source of various anti-cancer chemicals. Kale is very high in calcium, Vitamin A and iron. It is good for building up the calcium content of the body and builds strong teeth. Kale is beneficial to the digestive and nervous systems. It is protective against osteoporosis and bone loss disorders.

Medicinal Value of Whole Foods—CONTINUED

Lecithin: Protects the nerves and improves memory. Protects cells against damage by oxidation. Emulsifies fat in the blood. Helps to purify the liver.

Lemon: This citrus fruit ranks very high in its medicinal value, having many therapeutic uses. It is a good general blood and body purifier and a mild diuretic. The juice also aids in the removal of old drug poisons from the body.

Mushroom (maitake and shiitake): An immune enhancing longevity tonic, heart medicine and cancer remedy in Asia. Current tests show mushrooms, such as maitake, help prevent and/or treat cancer, viral diseases, high cholesterol, and high blood pressure. Eaten daily, maitake or shiitake, fresh (3 ounces) or dried (1/3 ounce), cut cholesterol by 7% to 12% respectively. Used to treat leukemia in China and breast cancer in Japan.

Nuts and Seeds: Nuts and seeds are endowed with a nearly complete array of vitamins and minerals. They are rich in protein of a high biological value. High in essential fatty-acids, which facilitate oxygen transport, assist proteins in building body cells, aid glandular activity, convert carotene into Vitamin A, and complement Vitamin D and calcium. The plant compounds in nuts have been shown to enhance immune functions and to help prevent chemically induced cancers. Nuts and seeds exhibit numerous anti-cancer effects. Nuts and seeds are excellent for chronic fatigue.

Olive oil: Easy to digest and imparts a generally soothing and healing influence to the digestive tract. Used therapeutically, it is beneficial for the gall bladder and liver. It strengthens and develops body tissue and is a tonic for the nerves. It helps to dissolve cholesterol deposits in the body.

Parsley: Anti-cancer proptertiers due to its high concentration of antioxidants. A blood builder and purifier. Good for stimulating bowel activity and brain activity. It is high in iron and rich in copper and manganese. It makes an excellent tea and helps to release retained water from the body.

Pineapple: Helps to detox the body. A main constituent of pineapple, *bromelain*, is an anti-inflammatory. The greatest value of pineapple lies in its digestive power, which closely resembles that of the human gastric juices. Pineapple helps to clear mucus waste from the bronchial tissues. It literally "digests" dead or diseased cells and foreign microbes in the throat.

Radish: Stimulates the appetite. Cleanses the gall bladder and helps expel stones. Helps to promote digestion and to remove mucus and phlegm from the body. Also help to cleanse the kidneys. Regular use helps to prevent viral infections such as the common cold and influenza.

Seaweed and Kelp: One of the best foods that you can eat to nourish the thyroid. Because seaweeds are so rich in minerals they help with many degenerative diseases. Benefits include reducing blood cholesterol and helping disorders of the genitourinary and reproductive systems. The iodine in seaweeds helps to prevent goiter and is indispensable to thyroid function. The thyroid influences digestive and metabolic efficiency. Kelp has anti-bacterial and anti-

Medicinal Value of Whole Foods—CONTINUED

viral activity. Most types of seaweed have anti-cancer activity. Studies conducted at McGill University in Canada have shown that some seaweeds (including arame, hiziki and kombu) can help remove radioactive elements from the body. Lastly, seaweeds have long been acclaimed as beauty aids, believed to help maintain beautiful healthy skin and lustrous hair.

Soybean: Rich in natural hormones. The anti-cancer activity is thought to be especially antagonistic to breast cancer, possibly one reason rates of breast and prostate cancers are low among the Japanese. Soybeans lower blood cholesterol substantially.

Spinach: Tops the list, along with other green leafy vegetables, as a food most eaten by people who don't get cancer. A super source of antioxidants and cancer antagonists, containing about four times more beta carotene and three times more lutein than broccoli. Rich in fiber, helps lower blood cholesterol. Eat raw or lightly cooked.

Spirulina: Called the miracle food, it is high in protein, Vitamin A, Vitamin B12, calcium, phosphorus, iron, magnesium and potassium. It is a blood builder and helps to detoxify the blood. It is also good for stamina and energy.

Swiss chard: Used to build energy. When mixed with carrot juice it helps to control urinary tract infections, hemorrhoids, skin diseases and constipation. A mild diuretic and laxative. It contains Vitamins A and C, potassium, calcium and iron.

Tomato: A major source of *lycopene*, an antioxidant and anti-cancer agent. Tomatoes are linked in particular to lower rates of pancreatic cancer and cervical cancer. Aids in the cleansing of toxins. Neutralizes uric acid from animal products and is good for digestive disorders. Avoid if you have arthritis.

Turmeric: Truly one of the marvelous medicinal spices of the world. Its main active ingredient is *curcumin* which gives turmeric its intense cadmium yellow color. Curcumin is an anti-inflammatory agent on a par with cortisone and has reduced symptoms of rheumatoid arthritis. It helps to lower cholesterol. It protects the liver from toxins, boosts stomach defenses against acid, lowers blood sugar in diabetics, and acts as a powerful antagonist of numerous cancer-causing agents.

Zucchini: A highly alkaline food that is an excellent remedy for acidosis of the liver and blood. It is high in minerals and low in calories making it a perfect food for weight loss. According to Chinese Medicine, squash helps to reduce inflammation.

REFERENCES

The Healing Power of Foods, by Michael Murray, N.D.

Food: Your Miracle Medicine, by Jean Carper

Healing Foods, by Patti Hausman, M.S.

The Good Fats and Oils, by Jean Barilla, M.S.

Medicinal Value of Natural Foods, by W.H. Graves, D.C.

Prescription for Dietary Wellness, by Phyllis Balch, C.N.C. and James Balch, M.D.

Whole Foods Companion, by Dianne Onstad

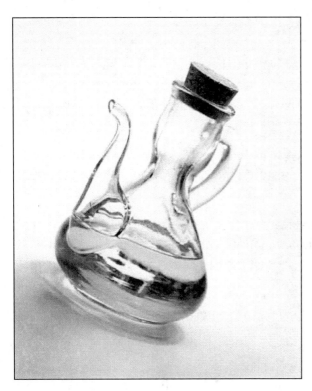

Confused About Fats?
Here's the Skinny
by Edward Bauman, M.Ed., Ph.D.

Our bodies create substances from fats that are necessary for good health — hence the term "essential fatty acids." Fat is used to store energy, make hormones, and transport vitamins, among other important functions. For a moderately active person, approximately one third of one's daily calories can come from healthy fats.

It is useful to think of fats as building blocks — and the better the blocks, the stronger the building. If there are only broken or damaged blocks available, you can still build a house, but the house won't have a strong foundation and eventually there will be problems.

Good Fats

Certain essential fatty acids are extremely beneficial. These include:

- ▶ Omega-3s,found in oily fish, algae, and some seeds and nuts;
- ▶ Omega-6s rich in GLA (gamma linolenic acid), found in evening primrose, borage, and red current oils;Omega 9s, found is olives, avocados, and nuts; and
- ▶ Uncooked saturated fats, found in coconut and raw dairy.

In our not so distant past, people consumed a healthy balance of oils and fats, which kept our immunity strong, our hormones in balance, our thinking clear, our energy even throughout the day, our skin, hair and eyes healthy, and even helped us maintain a healthy weight. Today, Americans consume large quantities of corrupted fats — found in packaged and processed foods, commercially baked goods, and fried foods — and not enough of the Omega-3 fats found in algae, fish, nuts, and seeds.

A general description of good fats is that they are naturally-occurring and haven't been damaged by high heat, refining, or over-processing. The best fats are found in:

- ▶ Fish (such as salmon and sardines)
- ▶ Nuts
- ▶ Avocados
- ▶ Seeds
- ▶ Fresh, organic creamery butter

- ▶ Cold-pressed extra-virgin olive oil
- ▶ Flaxseeds
- ▶ Organic whole milk products
- ▶ Organic eggs
- ▶ Coconut

Confused About Fats? Here's the Skinny—CONTINUED

Bad Fats

Saturated fats, which come mostly from animals — such as are found in butter, meats, and dairy products — have a bad reputation, but many nutrition experts believe it is not animal fat, per se, that is the problem, but the fact that they are usually refined, heated at high temperatures, or polluted by commercial farming methods. Due to abundant antibiotic and steroid use, fats from conventionally fed factory-farm animals should probably be consumed with caution, if at all.

"Bad fats" are damaged. They have become oxidized due to high heat processing, which removes healthy nutrients like Vitamin E and creates lipid compound that the body cannot utilize for healthy cell building.

Fats are often described as saturated, monounsaturated, or polyunsaturated. has All have different properties. In general, the monounsaturates (such as olive oil, avocado, and some nut oils) are good for you. We definitely need some saturated fats, but avoid those that have been exposed to high heat or chemical contamination, if possible. Polyunsaturates (especially in the form of refined vegetable oils) can be detrimental to your health over time, so choose a healthier fat when given a choice. Remember to read food labels, and avoid partially hydrogenated fats whenever you see them.

Here is a quick guide to the best and worst fats:

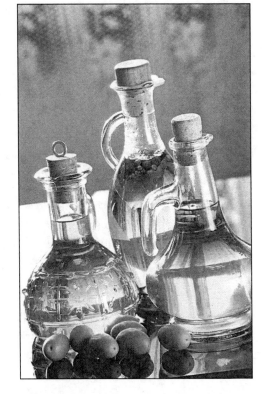

"Good" Fats "Bad" Fats

- ▶ Nuts
- ▶ Margarine
- ▶ Seeds
- ▶ Fried foods
- ▶ Avocados
- ▶ Partially hydro-genated fats
- ▶ Fish oils
- ▶ Refined vegetable oils
- ▶ Flaxseed oil and meal
- ▶ Saturated fats, in excess
- ▶ Olive oil and olives
- ▶ Most polyunsaturated fats
- ▶ Fresh butter (in moderation)

There is no need to be afraid of fat. Our bodies and brains require the healthy forms of fats in order to function well. Enjoy some good fats in your diet every day and you will reap their health benefits.

Acid-Alkaline Revisited

Studies at the Moffitt Hospital, University of California at San Francisco, have shown that the metabolism of certain foods either raises or lowers the concentration of acid and alkaline (base) in the blood. Fruits and vegetables add the alkaline bicarbonate ion to the blood, thus lowering the blood's acid level, while meat, poultry and fish produce acid, thereby raising blood acidity.

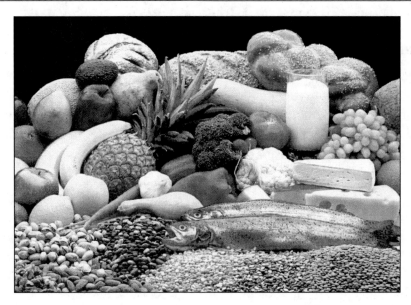

The modern diet, high in animal protein, creates more acid than base in the body, resulting in a "net acid load." Until recently, scientists thought that the kidneys safely excreted this excess acid, resulting in no undesirable physiological consequences. However, research now indicates that acid can be retained in the body, and its presence is linked to osteoporosis, loss of muscle mass, and reduction of hormone levels — all symptoms associated with aging. Declining kidney efficiency is common as people age, and contributes to the problem of acid buildup. Renal tubular failure may eventually result.

Researchers recommend that people modify their diets as they age to reduce the net acid loads. This means cutting down on animal foods. By putting more vegetables into their diets, people may reduce their chances of developing osteoporosis, kidney disease, and other age-related problems.

Considerable attention is now focused on the role of calcium in osteoporosis, but too much acid caused by high-protein diets may be the true villain. In one study, women whose net acid load was neutralized by alkaline supplements experienced increased retention of calcium and phosphorus, and greater new bone formation.

Based on *Consumers' Research,* Dec 1997.

Alkaline Forming, Neutral & Acid Forming Foods

ALKALINE FORMING FOODS	NEUTRAL FOODS	ACID FORMING FOODS
Beans (sprouted)	Almonds	Beans (dried)
Buckwheat	Avocado	Bread
Fruit	Brazil nuts	Cashews
Herbs (green)	Butter	Coffee
Millet	Cheese (goat)	Cranberries
Nuts (soaked)	Coconut	Eggs
Quinoa	Corn	Flour (refined)
Seaweed	Cruciferous family	Meats
Seeds (sprouted)	Flax seed	Milk (pasteurized products)
Vegetables (leafy and raw)	Hemp seed	Oats
	Honey	Peanuts
	Milk (non-fat products)	Peas (dried)
	Milk (raw products)	Pecans
	Oil (vegetable)	Pomegranates
	Pumpkin seeds	Poultry
	Rice (brown)	Rice (white)
	Sesame seed	Rye
	Sunflower seed	Seafood
		Strawberries
		Sugar (refined)
		Tofu
		Wheat

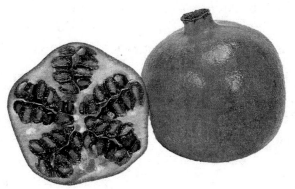

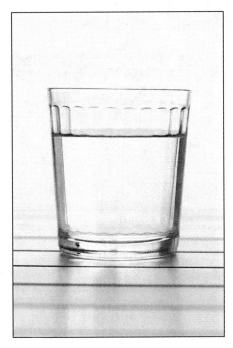

The Role of Pure Water in Detoxification

by Robert M. Vineyard

There are more than 3800 chemicals in daily use, many of which make their way into our drinking water. Less than half of these have been tested for toxic effects in humans, and less than 10% have been tested for toxicity in children. The *National Institute of Health* (NIH) recently estimated our polluted environment accounts for 50% of cancer risk.

In recent years, the role of heavy metals and xenobiotics (pesticides, herbicides, and industrial wastes) as causes of a wide variety of adverse health effects is receiving more and more attention. These accumulating toxins are insidious and prevalent agents capable of interfering with physiologic functions of all human systems. One cannot expect the normal detoxification systems of the body to function optimally when these substances are constantly present. In fact, the body's ability to remove these substances becomes diminished and they are in turn stored in adipose tissues.

With the growing awareness that environmental pollutants have crept into every corner of the food chain and our water supplies, many health care professionals are encouraging patients to undergo detoxification regimes. These programs encourage the body to unload its stores of accumulated environmental toxins.

Surprisingly, many of these programs fail to mention the role of pure water in detoxification. Through years of research regarding the role water plays within our bodies, it was thought that water had four functions: a solvent, transportant, lubricant, and coolant. The fifth function, that of an electro-negative enhancer, is a relatively new concept discovered through subsequent studies that revealed when water is consumed in its purest form (H_2O and nothing else), it has remarkable and unique benefits for our health.

As the body ingests foods, water contributes in the breakdown and absorption of nutrients and is a key element in the removal of wastes. During detoxification, wastes that have been stored in adipose tissues are dumped into the bloodstream and lymph, and then sent to the liver and kidneys for processing and elimination. Here is where water's fifth function, that of electro-negative enhancer, comes into play: by optimizing the natural space between red blood cells, which reduces the risk of heart disease by helping to avoid clotting; and by allowing the fat cell to detox by off-loading metabolic wastes and environmental toxins into the bloodstream for elimination. This also assists in weight loss and reduces water retention.

To understand this we must understand the characteristics of the *adipose cell*. It is a function of the fat cell to store what the body cannot use and/or get rid of. An adipose cell contains for the most part salts, sugars, tiny amounts of lipid, and other organic pollutants, all bathed in an ocean of water. These salts and heavy metal inorganics have an affinity for others, a magnetic attraction so to speak. Fat cells

The Role of Pure Water in Detoxification—CONTINUED

are good not bad. They store toxic material and keep it from being deposited in vital areas. However, when the fat cell has reached its limit of storage, it will allow the deposition of metabolites and wastes in other areas, such as the blood vessels.

Ingestion of copious quantities of pure water enhances the electro-negativity. Through osmosis, the fat cell will try to take in more of this pure water. Because the water is pure, the fat cell will disperse its contents into solution and those contents will be removed through the kidneys more readily because of the volume and ability pure water has to carry wastes.

However, this fifth function is diminished when we drink water containing high concentrations of dissolved minerals and contaminants. The minerals found in spring and mineral water are inorganic. They are not in a form that can be easily assimilated by the human body. True, we all need minerals to maintain healthy living, but they must be of an organic origin. Humans do not have enzymes to digest rock, or we could obtain necessary minerals by sucking on stones. Simply put: plants (and microbes in the soil) eat rocks, and we eat plants.

Our kidneys filter 400 gallons of fluid each day. If there is enough water present, kidneys operate easily. If not, kidneys are forced to recycle too much and deposits may be left behind in the form of stones. Many of a kidney stone's mineral constituents are the same as those found in tap water or bottled spring water.

Water is a poor source for dietary minerals due to the incredible variance in quantity and blend. For example, to obtain any meaningful contribution to your dietary intake of calcium you would have to consume more than five gallons of water per day. Recognizing that most people don't consume the old standard of eight glasses per day, we can see that counting on water as a source of minerals is foolish.

If water carries a load of mineral salts, heavy metals, and pollutants, then it cannot be efficient in its vital functions. If your car has rusty water in the radiator, it overheats. If we have an abnormal waste level in our blood, we overheat and develop fever. This is why during detoxification it is not uncommon to feel ill and feverish; the body is dumping the stored toxins into solution so they can be removed.

Water that is void of organic contaminants and dissolved inorganic rocks is the type of water we need to consume. Drinking at least two liters of pure water daily will improve the roles that water plays within our bodies through its ability to move nutrients deeply into tissues, pick up wastes, keep us cool, and maintain joints without leaving deposits.

Robert Vineyard is president and founder of *Pure Water Systems, Inc.* where they manufacture the *PWStm BEV-Series* in-home pure water appliances. Combining three different purification technologies, the BEV-Series systems produce 100% pure, contaminant-free drinking water. For more information on water testing and innovative technology advances, call **866-444-9926** or visit online at: **www.purewatersystems.com**

Tonic Teas: Herbal Teas as Healing Beverages

by Edward Bauman, M.Ed., Ph.D.

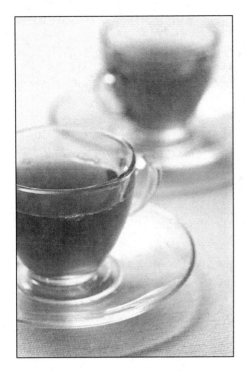

Herbal teas have been used as healing beverages since the beginning of time. They were initially wildcrafted by observant folk healers who noticed the beneficial effects plants had on the sick or aging animals who ate them.

The following therapeutic teas can be consumed in quantities of 2 to 4 cups a day to add valuable trace minerals to the diet that will help overcome the wear and tear of age, stress, illness, injury, medications, and a history of less than optimal foods. A teaspoon per cup of raw honey can be added if the taste is too earthy for you to enjoy.

Please consult with a certified herbalist or nutritional professional if you need more information and support.

RECIPES

All recipes call for dried herbs. For the best quality and best prices, seek out a natural food store or specialty shop that sells organic herbs and spices in bulk.

Calcium Tea

GOOD FOR MENSTRUAL, MUSCLE, INTESTINAL CRAMPS, HEART, AND NERVES.

Add 2 tablespoons of each herb per quart of water. Steep in boiled water for 20 to 30 minutes.

Chamomile

Comfrey

Borage

Oat straw

Emotional Stabilizer

A DRINK FOR OVERWROUGHT AND STRESSED-OUT FOLKS. (DO NOT USE LICORICE IF YOU HAVE HIGH BLOOD PRESSURE OR ARE PREGNANT!)

Add 2 tablespoons of each herb per quart of water. Steep in boiled water for 20 to 30 minutes.

Oat straw

Elecampane

Kelp

Comfrey

Rosemary

Eucalyptus leaves

Licorice or Star Anise

Mint

Tonic Teas: Herbal Teas as Healing Beverages—CONTINUED

Hot Toddy *(4 servings)*

(DO NOT USE LICORICE IF YOU HAVE HIGH BLOOD PRESSURE OR ARE PREGNANT!)

Bring to a boil: 1 quart unfiltered apple juice. Add 1 teaspoon of 3 of the following herbs and steep for 30-45 minutes.

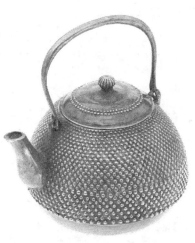

Sarsaparilla
Licorice
Hibiscus
Sassafras
Star Anise
Lemon grass
Cinnamon stick
Ginger

Trace Elements Tea

VERY SOOTHING TO THE NERVOUS SYSTEM, AND HELPS ALKALINIZE AN OVERSTRESSED BODY.

Add 2 tablespoons of each herb per quart of water. Steep in boiled water for 20 to 30 minutes.

Alfalfa
Fennel
Seaweed
Nettle
Watercress
Slippery elm

Intestinal Tea *(4 servings)*

THIS TEA IS ALKALINIZING, COOLING, AND NUTRITIOUS. SPICY!

To one quart of Trace Elements Tea (above) add:

1 Tbsp. fresh-squeezed lemon juice
1 Tbsp. brewer's yeast
1 Tbsp. rosehip powder
1-2 tsp. cayenne pepper
1+ tsp. paprika
6 oz. spring water if you care to dilute this further
Optional: 1+ tsp. bee pollen and/or honey

Iron Tea

EVEN POPEYE WOULD APPROVE OF THIS ONE. SUPER CLEANSING FOR YOUR LIVER, TOO!

Add 2 tablespoons of each herb per quart of water. Steep in boiled water for 20 to 30 minutes.

Yellow dock
Watercress
Dandelion root
Nettle
Parsley
Dulse

Mellow Beverage Teas

IT'S FUN TO MAKE YOUR OWN HERBAL TEA BLENDS.

Combine these herbs in different proportions to create tasty new teas. Add 2 tablespoons of each herb per quart of water. Steep in boiled water for 20 to 30 minutes.

Mint
Chamomile
Raspberry leaves
Yarrow
Papaya leaves
Lemon grass
Rosehips
Red clover
Sage
Lemon verbena
Hibiscus
Basil

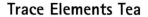

Excerpted with permission from *Recipes and Remedies for Rejuvenation,* ©2005 by Edward Bauman, M.Ed., Ph.D., published by Bauman College, Penngrove, CA. To learn more from Dr. Ed Bauman, visit **www.baumancollege.org**

Reactive Food Families

FOOD FAMILY	MEMBERS OF FAMILY
Apple	Apple, pear, and quince.
Banana	Banana, arrowroot, and plantain.
Buckwheat	Buckwheat, rhubarb, and sorrel.
Cane	Cane sugar and molasses.
Chocolate	Chocolate and cocoa.
Citrus	Grapefruit, lemon, lime, tangerine, kumquat, and orange.
Composite flower	Lettuce, endive, chicory, escarole, artichoke, and dandelion.
Corn	Corn, blue corn, and popcorn.
Crustacean	Crab, shrimp, lobster, and crayfish.
Dairy	All foods derived from cow's milk: milk, cheese, yogurt, cottage cheese.
Fish	Trout, tuna, halibut, red snapper, sole, salmon, sardine, haddock, smelt, whitefish, mahi-mahi, flounder, herring, petrale, scrod, and steelhead.
Fungi	Mushrooms, brewer's and baker's yeast.
Gluten grain	Wheat, rye, oats, spelt, kamut, and barley.
Goosefoot	Beet, spinach, chard, and Swiss chard.
Grape	Grape, raisin, and buckthorn tea.
Heath	Blueberry, cranberry, and huckleberry.
Honey	Honey, bee pollen, and royal jelly.
Laurel	Avocado and bay leaf.
Legume	Beans and peas, alfalfa, green bean, lentils, black-eyed pea, peanut, and licorice.

FOOD FAMILY	MEMBERS OF FAMILY
Lily	Asparagus, onion, garlic, chive, green onion, leek, scallion, shallot, and aloe vera.
Mollusk	Clam, oyster, scallop, mussel, squid, and abalone.
Morning glory	Sweet potato and yam.
Mustard and cruciferous	Mustard, cabbage, collard greens, cauliflower, broccoli, Brussels sprouts, turnip, kale, rutabaga, kohlrabi, radish, horseradish, and watercress.
Nightshade	Potato, tomato, eggplant, bell peppers, red peppers, green peppers, chilis, cayenne pepper, tomatillo, pimiento, and tobacco.
Olive	Green and black olives.
Papaya	Papaya
Parsley	Parsley, parsnip, carrot, celery, caraway, anise, dill, fennel, coriander, and cilantro.
Pineapple	Pineapple
Plum	Plum, prune, cherry, almond, nectarine, apricot, and peach.
Poultry	Chicken, turkey, capon, grouse, duck, pheasant, goose, and partridge.
Rice	White, brown and basmati rice.
Rose	Strawberry, blackberry, loganberry, and raspberry.
Sunflower	Sunflower, Jerusalem artichoke, and safflower.
Walnut	Walnut, butternut, hickory nut, and pecan.

Most Commonly Reactive Foods From "The False Fat Diet," by Elson Haas, M.D

The Sensitive Seven

1. Dairy
2. Wheat
3. Corn
4. Eggs
5. Soy
6. Peanuts
7. Sugar

The Other Usual Suspects

▶ Additives, dyes, sulfites, and preservatives
▶ Aspartame
▶ Beer
▶ Chocolate
▶ Citrus fruits
▶ Cocktail mixes
▶ Coffee
▶ Crab
▶ Gluten: wheat, rye, barley, oats, spelt, and kamut
▶ MSG
▶ Oats
▶ Potatoes
▶ Rye
▶ Shellfish
▶ Shrimp
▶ Tomatos
▶ Wine
▶ Yeast

Occasionally Reactive Foods

▶ Bacon and other pork products
▶ Bananas
▶ Barley
▶ Beef
▶ Berries
▶ Black pepper
▶ Celery
▶ Cherries
▶ Chicken
▶ Coconut
▶ Grapes
▶ Kidney beans
▶ Melon
▶ Mushrooms
▶ Mustard
▶ Nuts
▶ Onions
▶ Peas
▶ Pineapple
▶ Plums
▶ Quinoa
▶ Raisins
▶ Spices: cloves, curry, turmeric, and cinnamon
▶ Strawberries
▶ Vinegar

THE GOOD GUYS: Foods That Are Seldom Reactive

▶ Apricots
▶ Beets
▶ Broccoli
▶ Cabbage
▶ Carrots
▶ Cauliflower
▶ Cranberries
▶ Halibut
▶ Honey
▶ Kale
▶ Lamb
▶ Olives
▶ Olive oil
▶ Pears
▶ Rabbit
▶ Rice
▶ Salmon
▶ Sole
▶ Squash
▶ Sweet potatoes
▶ Tapioca
▶ Trout
▶ Turkey

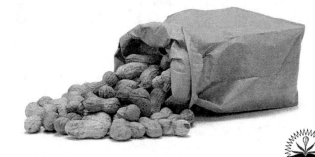

What is Your Diet Direction?

by Edward Bauman, M.Ed., Ph.D.

Establishing a diet direction is a way to organize the amounts and varieties of foods one chooses to consume in order to achieve a specific effect. Like life, diet directions change over time, sometimes intentionally, sometimes impulsively. The three main diet directions are:

- ▶ Building
- ▶ Balancing
- ▶ Cleansing

The benefits of following each of these three diet directions are discussed below. The length of time one follows a designated diet direction depends on his or her health status.

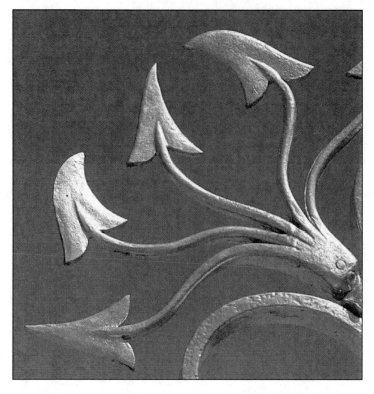

It is common for a person to follow a cleansing diet for three to 14 days at a time, a balancing diet for 14-21 days, and a building diet for 21-42 days. A building diet program is typically longer in duration because most people who need this kind of help are tired, nutrient depleted, and have a long history of eating poor-quality foods

Building Diet

Many people with chronic immune system disorders, carbohydrate cravings, and excess weight feel better if they follow a diet that includes fewer carbohydrates and more protein and fats. A *Building Diet* is comprised of a higher percentage of calories from protein and fats relative to carbohydrates.

The Zone Diet is a building diet, with its formula of 30% calories from protein, 30% calories from fats, and 40% calories from carbohydrates. The Atkins Diet, a high-protein, high-fat, limited-carbohydrate diet, is another type of building diet — albeit not a very healthy one.

Building diets are appropriate for people who are growing rapidly, like children and teenagers, as well as competitive athletes, adults doing manual labor, or those recovering from illness or injury. It is crucial that a person on a building diet eat ample amounts of fresh vegetables (5 servings per day) and fruits (2 to 3 servings per day) and drink herbal teas rather than caffeinated beverages to maintain a healthy acid-alkaline (pH) balance.

What is Your Diet Direction?—CONTINUED

Balancing Diet

A *Balancing Diet* is comprised of equal amounts of protein and fats relative to carbohydrates. A prudent application of the USDA Food Pyramid by the *Cancer and Heart Association* is an example of this approach.

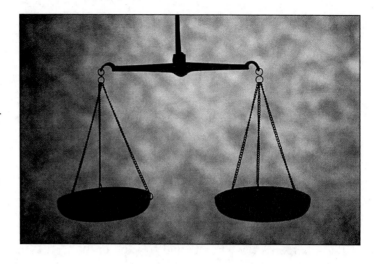

A balanced diet would include a wide variety of healthy foods and would typically supply 20% of calories from protein, 30% of calories from fat, and 50% of calories from carbohydrates. The key to this approach is that the foods be seasonal, local, and organic whenever possible. The Balancing Diet in the *Eating For Health*™ approach is quite different than the so-called "balanced diet" advised by industry-driven nutritionists and dieticians.

Many people today are confused about carbohydrates, thinking they are all bad. In fact, complex carbohydrates are an essential part of the diet. It is refined carbohydrates in the form of flour and sugar that wreak havoc on one's health. The health-promoting complex carbs include grains, vegetables, and fruits.

Eating For Health™ suggests using whole, non-glutinous grains, such as rice, millet, and quinoa, as staple grains in lieu of the traditionally over-consumed and more allergenic wheat, corn, oats, and rye. Roughly equal amounts of fruits and vegetables may be consumed, with an emphasis on eating whole fruits rather than juice or fruit products made from concentrates, to moderate the amount of sugar the body will have to metabolize at one sitting.

Cleansing Diet

A *Cleansing Diet* will consist of more calories from carbohydrates (>60%) relative to proteins (20%) and fats (<20%). This is a fat-sparing, adequate-protein, high-complex carbohydrate, low-glycemic (sugar content) diet. The Ornish, Weil, McDougall, and hypoallergenic diets are all in this category.

The main objective is to lower the fat content while maintaining adequate protein and increasing the amount of fruits and vegetables in the diet. Dairy products would also be eliminated due to their mucous-forming properties. Proteins from vegetable sources such as legumes, seeds, nuts, and marine algae would be preferred over meat, eggs, fish, or fowl.

Maintaining an alkaline-forming diet by including generous amounts of fresh fruits and vegetables, as well as their juices, with the addition of chlorophyll-rich foods like herbs and micro-green powders, would replenish the minerals that are commonly missing from a non-plant-based diet.

What is Your Diet Direction?—CONTINUED

Using a Diet Direction Effectively

The key to successfully applying a diet direction is to build the food plan on top-quality whole foods. Food quality is diminished in most commercial restaurants and with most packaged food items. Fresh is always best.

One's diet direction is a reminder to eat more of certain kinds of foods, such as nuts and seeds in a building diet, and less of other foods, such as bread products in a cleansing diet. Having an intention to eat well helps a person decide what to eat and what to pass up. Cookies, candy, ice cream, sodas, and foods with artificial colors, flavors, and preservatives are best left on the shelves, no matter one's diet direction.

As individuals become more conscious with their food choices, they are more in touch with how certain combinations of foods feel to them. At certain times of the day, when hunger hits and hits quickly, such a person knows what food to keep on hand tosatisfy hunger while providing nourishing energy. Almonds and raisins are more nourishing than a Milky Way, and the energy that is produced clears the brain and mobilizes the body into action.

Eating For Health™ is a skill that is learned with the support of a food coach who can serve as a mentor and resource. Replacing depleting foods in the diet with health-promoting ones is a gradual process, but one new food per week will increase a person's repertoire by four foods per month, or 48 foods per year.

What about parties or a food craving that just won't quit? It is fine to socialize occasionally with special food and drink. It is what we consume habitually that makes or breaks our health. The key is to not be too hungry or tired before a big occasion, or else overeating and excessive drinking may prevail.

Proper food choices provide a strong nutritional foundation for life, help protect us from the health challenges we encounter, and allow us to live up to our potential as dynamic, creative human beings.

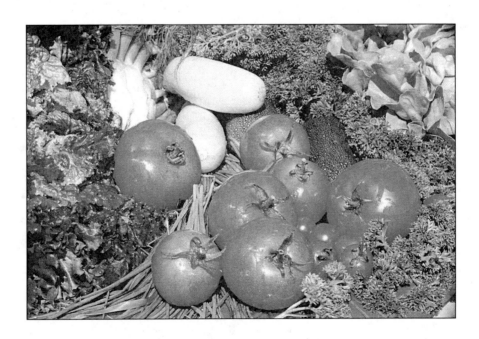

The Essential EatingWell™ Seafood Guide

Best Choices

FISH OR SEAFOOD	HEALTH CONCERNS	OMEGA-35	HARVEST NOTES
Anchovies	No advisory	RICH	Abundant
Catfish (farmed)	No advisory	Modest	Environmentally benign
Caviar (U.S. farmed)	No advisory	RICH	Environmentally benign
Clams	No advisory	Modest	Abundant
Cod (Pacific)	No advisory	Modest	Abundant
Crab (except King and Blue)	Mercury contamination: limit to 1 meal/week	Modest	Abundant
Flounder (Pacific)	No advisory	Modest	Abundant
Halibut (Pacific)	Mercury contamination: limit to 2 meals/month	Good	Abundant
Herring	No advisory	RICH	Abundant
Mackerels (except King)	No advisory	RICH	Abundant
Mahi Mahi (Dorado)	Mercury contamination: limit to 1 meal/week	Modest	Abundant
Mussels	No advisory	Good	Abundant
Oysters	No advisory	Modest	Environmentally benign
Pollock (Pacific)	PCB residues: limit to 1 meal/week	Good	Abundant
Salmon (wild)	No advisory	RICH	Well managed (some endangered)
Sardines	No advisory	RICH	Abundant
Shrimp (U.S. farmed, U.S. or Canadian wild caught)	No advisory	Good	Abundant/Environmentally benign
Sole (Pacific, English Dover)	No advisory	Modest	Abundant
Squids	No advisory	Good	Abundant
Striped Bass (farmed)	No advisory	Very Good	Environmentally benign
Sturgeon (farmed)	No advisory	RICH	Environmentally benign
Tilapia (farmed, U.S. and Central America)	No advisory	Modest	Environmentally benign (U.S.), ecologically destructive (foreign)
Trout (Rainbow, farmed)	No advisory	Very Good	Environmentally benign

The Essential EatingWell™ Seafood Guide—CONTINUED

Best Choices (continued)

FISH OR SEAFOOD	HEALTH CONCERNS	OMEGA-35	HARVEST NOTES
Tuna (canned, light)	No advisory	Modest	Abundant
Tuna (yellowfin, farmed)	Mercury contamination: limit to 3 meals/month	Good	Environmentally benign

Caution Advised

FISH OR SEAFOOD	HEALTH CONCERNS	OMEGA-35	HARVEST NOTES
Crab (King)	No advisory	Modest	Regionally overfished
Lobster (Maine/American)	Mercury contamination: limit to 2 meals/month	Modest	Regionally overfished
Lobster (spiny/rock)	No advisory	Modest	Regionally overfished
Monkfish	Mercury contamination: limit to 2 meals/month	Modest	Overfished
Oysters (wild)	PCB residues: limit to 3 meals/month	Very good	Abundant
Salmon (farmed)	PCB, dioxin and pesticide residues: limit to less than 1 meal/month	RICH	Farms are ecologically destructive
Scallops	No advisory	Modest	Abundant/Regionally overfished
Sea Bass (wild)	Mercury contamination: limit to 1 meal/week	Very good	Abundant
Tuna (canned, white)	Mercury contamination: limit to 3 meals/month	Very good	Abundant
Tuna (steaks)	Mercury contamination: limit to 1 meal/month	Very good	Abundant

Worst Choices

FISH OR SEAFOOD	HEALTH CONCERNS	OMEGA-35	HARVEST NOTES
Bluefish	PCB, mercury and pesticide contamination: Avoid	Very good	Overfished
Caviar (wild sturgeon)	No advisory	RICH	Severely overfished
Chilean Sea Bass	Mercury contamination: limit to 2 meals/month	Very good	Severely overfished Destructive harvest

The Essential EatingWell™ Seafood Guide—CONTINUED

Worst Choices (continued)

FISH OR SEAFOOD	HEALTH CONCERNS	OMEGA-35	HARVEST NOTES
Cod (Atlantic)	No advisory	Modest	Severely overfished
Crab (blue)	Mercury contamination, PCB residues: limit to 1 meal/month	Good	Recovering
Flounder (Atlantic)	No advisory	Modest	Severely overfished
Grouper	Mercury contamination: limit to 1 meal/month	Modest	Severely overfished
Haddock	No advisory	Modest	Severely overfished/Recovering
Halibut (Atlantic)	Mercury contamination, PCB residues: limit to 2 meals/month	Good	Severely overfished
Mackerel (king)	High levels of mercury contamination: Avoid	RICH	Abundant
Marlin	High levels of mercury contamination: Avoid	Modest	Severely overfished
Orange Roughy	Mercury contamination: limit to 1 meal/month	Modest	Severely overfished Destructive harvest
Pacific Rockfish (snapper)	Mercury contamination: limit to 1 meal/month	Good	Severely overfished
Sharks	High levels of mercury contamination: Avoid	RICH	Destructive harvest
Shrimp (wild, foreign)	No advisory	Good	Destructive harvest
Snapper (red)	Mercury contamination: limit to 1 meal/month	Good	Severely overfished Destructive harvest
Sole (Atlantic)	PCB residues: limit to 1 meal/month	Modest	Severely overfished Destructive harvest
Swordfish	High levels of mercury contamination: Avoid	Very Good	Regionally overfished
Tilefish	High levels of mercury contamination: Avoid	Good	Severely overfished
Tuna (bluefin)	Mercury contamination: limit to 1 meal/month	RICH	Severely overfished Destructive harvest

SOURCES:
Environmental Defense/Oceans Alive, Linus Pauling Institute, Seafood Watch, Monterey Bay Aquarium

Notes

_____
_____
_____
_____
_____
_____
_____
_____
_____
_____
_____
_____
_____
_____
_____
_____
_____
_____
_____
_____
_____
_____
_____

PART THREE:
Choosing & Growing the Best Organic Foods

Going organic begins with appreciating what these superior foods bring to our cells, which is vital nutrition and pure pleasure combined. Many people question the value of purchasing organic foods on a regular basis. It is true that, in most cases, organic foods are more expensive than their commercial counterparts. But cost does not equal value. If the organic foods are superior in terms of taste and nutritional value, then there is no doubt that they give you more value for your food dollar.

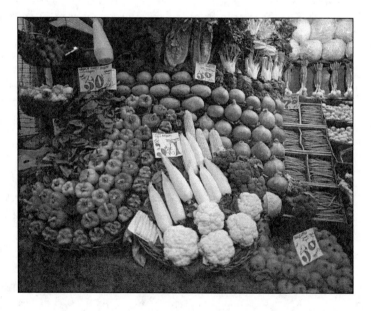

Organic foods tend to be significantly higher in essential minerals and substantially lower in toxic pesticides, herbicides, fungicides, waxes, and sprays than conventionally raised foods. Many people find that they taste better, too.

Of course, for best taste and nutritional value, organic foods should be eaten as close as possible to the time of harvest. Organic foods spoil much more quickly then commercial foods because chemicals are not used to extend their shelf life. Don't pay less for old and soggy organic foods that have been marked down before they rot. Look for the brightest and best organic foods in season, when their prices will be lowest. You can freeze, dry, or home can some seasonal foods to enjoy their benefits all through the winter months.

Introduction—CONTINUED

Please learn which foods are the least and the most contaminated and steer away from the latter. Foods that are waxed and sprayed can cause aggravations in the digestive, respiratory, hepatic, gastrointestinal, and immune systems. By eating poor-quality, non-organic foods, we rob our cells of vital nutrients and create a state of poor health and increased toxicity that can lead to diminished performance, mood, and energy, and eventually very expensive medical care. Considering all this, does it seem worth saving a dollar to buy non-organic food?

I suggest that everyone assess the percentage of organic food they are currently eating and increase it by 10% or more each month. In this way, folks are not overwhelmed by the seemingly high cost of the food as they begin to notice that the more organic food they eat, the better they feel. Similarly, buying more organic food will eventually bring down prices — the principle of supply and demand at work.

Growing your own organic food is the very best way to insure freshness and protect against food irradiation, gassing, coloring, and genetically modified organisms. Start with a window box of herbs, then drop some vegetable starts into a corner of the yard in summer, such as tomatoes, green beans, and squash. Create a salad garden of micro-greens; in some areas, it will produce all year long. Finally, buy some berry bushes and fruit trees that grow well in your area. In just a couple of years, you will be reaping what you have sown. Many areas offer community garden plots for people who do not have a yard in which to plant organic foods.

Gardening is far easier than you might think and will provide you with a wonderful outdoor hobby. The more produce you grow organically, the more you will have to share with your family and friends. Who knows, you might even have enough to sell at the farmers market.

What a delight, to care for your own growing crops! Being in the garden is the perfect recovery after a hard day on the road or at the office. The air in the garden smells so sweet. The plants have a way of speaking to you as you tend to them. "More water, please." "A little natural fertilizer would be great!" "Thank you so much for your love and care."

What a difference it makes to appreciate foods as the source of life and to therefore choose the best, rather than feeding ourselves and our families foods that have been processed, packaged, frozen, microwaved, and eaten on the run — without giving the least thought to their origin or nature.

What is Organic?

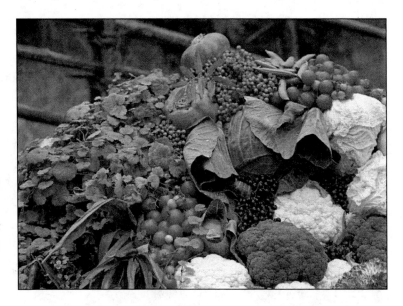

The word "organic" refers to both a philosophy and a system of production that mirrors the natural laws of living organisms, with an emphasis on the interdependence of all life. Applying the wisdom of generations, organic farmers care for the health of the land, the animals, and the people who eat their food. They recognize the interdependence of all life and the value of sustainability, which results in the highest quality and purest foods possible.

Industry definition of Organic

On October 21, 2002, new regulations went into effect governing the labeling of foods that are produced using organic agriculture. Here are the major points of these regulations:

▶ The use of irradiation, sewage sludge, or genetically modified organisms is prohibited in organic production;

▶ Antibiotic and synthetic hormone use is prohibited in the raising of organic meat and poultry, and 100% organic feed is required for organic livestock;

▶ The *National Organic Standards Board's* recommendations govern which substances are allowed or prohibited in the production and processing of organic foods; and

▶ Only food products that contain 95-100% certified organic ingredients may use the USDA seal.

What do national standards mean for consumers?

For consumers who want to minimize personal exposure to toxins and support humane and sustainable agricultural practices, the organic labeling laws are extremely important. Today, all agricultural products labeled "organic" have been verified by an accredited certification agency as meeting or exceeding USDA standards for organic production.

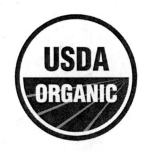

Adapted from *Organic Trade Association,* www.ota.com

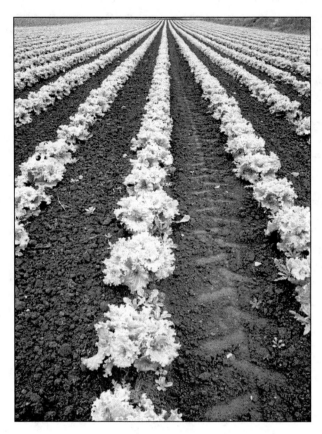

Research Brief...

Scientists Estimate That Pesticides Are Reducing Crop Yields by One-Third Through Impaired Nitrogen Fixation

Jennifer E. Fox, Jay Gulledge, Erika Engelhaupt, Matthew E. Burrow, and John A. McLachlan. Proceedings of the National Academy of Sciences, Vol. 104, No. 24, June 12, 2007

Over the last forty years nitrogen fertilizer use has increased seven-fold and nearly every acre of intensively farmed, conventional cropland is treated with pesticides. A team of scientists explored the impact of pesticides and other environmental toxicants on *symbiotic nitrogen fixation* (SNF) brought about by Rhizobium bacteria (Fox et al., 2007).

The team describes the critical role played by SNF in supporting crop yields and environmental quality. SNF has great potential to reduce farm production costs — a factor of growing importance as rising natural gas prices push upward the cost of nitrogen fertilizers. In Brazil, SNF from soybeans reduces production costs an estimated $1.3 billion per year. The research by Fox et al. (2007) explored in depth the signaling processes between plants and bacteria colonizing plant roots — processes that govern the degree of SNF and the production of certain phytochemicals. They focused on the ways that pesticides can disrupt signaling and impair the efficiency of SNF. Some 30 pesticides are known to disrupt SNF; the most widely used pesticide in the United States, glyphosate (Roundup) is known to be toxic to nitrogen fixing bacteria.

The "Conclusions" section of the paper begins by stating:

"The results of this study demonstrate that one of the environmental impacts of pesticides and contaminants in the soil environment is disruption of chemical signaling between the host plants and N-fixing Rhiz(obia) necessary for efficient SNF and optimal plant yield."

Drawing on their recent work and other published studies, the team projected that pesticides and other contaminants are reducing plant yield by one-third as a result of impaired SNF. This remarkable conclusion suggests one mechanism, or explanation of the yield-enhancing benefits of well-managed, long-term organic farming systems.

How to Get Organic Milk Into Your Kids' School

by Elaine Marie Lipson

from www.organicvalley.coop

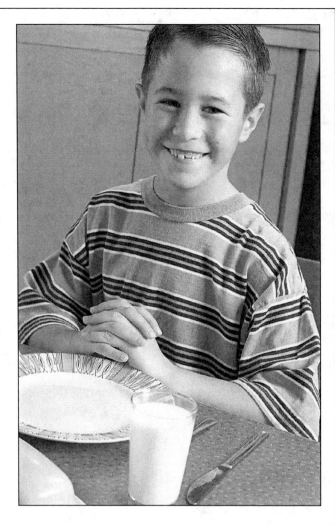

You're a caring, concerned parent — and if you could, you'd probably personally oversee every meal your child eats. Instead, you send them off to school each day hoping they'll make the best possible choices in the cafeteria or at the vending machine.

Milk is an especially important choice, and some schools are eliminating sodas and making milk more available to kids. That's an important step. But if you're one of many parents who chooses organic milk at home, perhaps you'd like to see your children have that choice in school, too.

Why not work to make that happen? You and other like-minded parents can influence what schools purchase and sell, not just in the lunchroom but also in vending machines, as "a lá carte" items, and at special events. The *Parents' Organic Toolkit* (found at **www.organicvalley.coop**) will help you get started, as you inform other parents about your mission, gather community support, and talk to the professionals at your children's schools about organic milk.

Where can your school use organic milk?

- ▶ Vending machines
- ▶ Special events
- ▶ Lunchroom
- ▶ Food service and cafeteria recipes
- ▶ Field trips

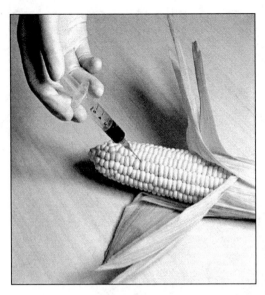

Genetically Engineered Foods: A Source of Rising Food Allergies?

Jeffrey M. Smith, Author of Seeds of Deception and Genetic Roulette • www.Responsibletechnology.org/

The huge jump in childhood food allergies in the US is in the news often.[1] But most reports fail to consider a link to a recent radical change in America's diet.

Beginning in 1996, bacteria, virus and other genes have been artificially inserted to the DNA of soy, corn, cottonseed and canola plants. These unlabeled *genetically modified* (GM) foods carry a risk of triggering life-threatening allergic reactions.

Evidence collected over the past decade now suggests that they are contributing to higher allergy rates. Scientists have long known that GM crops might cause allergies, but there are no tests to prove in advance that a GM crop is safe.[2] That's because people aren't usually allergic to a food until they have eaten it several times. According to former FDA microbiologist Louis Pribyl:

"The only definitive test for allergies," "is human consumption by affected peoples, which can have ethical considerations."[3]

And it is the ethical considerations of feeding unlabeled, high-risk GM crops to unknowing consumers that have many people up in arms.

UK Experiences Alarming Rise in Soy-Related Food Allergies

The UK is one of the few countries conducting a yearly evaluation of food allergies. In March 1999, researchers at the York Laboratory were alarmed to discover that reactions to soy have skyrocketed by 50% over the previous year.

Genetically modified soy had recently entered the UK from U.S. imports. So the soy used in the study was largely GM. John Graham, spokesman for the York laboratory, said, "We believe this raises serious new questions about the safety of GM foods."[4]

Critics of GM foods often say that the U.S. population is being used as guinea pigs in an experiment. But experiments have the benefit of controls and measurement. In this case, there is neither.

GM food safety experts point out that even if someone tried to collect data about allergic reactions to GM foods, they would likely be unsuccessful. "The potential allergen is rarely identified. The number of allergy-related medical visits is not tabulated. Even repeated visits due to well-known allergens are not counted as part of any established surveillance system."[5]

Indeed, the Canadian government announced in 2002 that they would "keep a careful eye on the health of Canadians"[6] to see if GM foods had any adverse reactions. They abandoned their plans within a year, saying that such a study was too difficult.

Genetically Engineered Foods: A Source of Rising Food Allergies?—CONTINUED

Creating New Proteins in a Lab — Good For Your Health?

The classical understanding of why a GM crop might create new allergies is that the imported genes produce a brand new protein. The novel protein may trigger reactions.

This was demonstrated in the mid 1990s when soybeans were outfitted with a gene from the Brazil nut. Scientists attempted to produce a healthier soybean, but ended up with a potentially deadly one. Blood tests from people who were allergic to Brazil nuts showed reactions to the beans.[7] Fortunately, this soy never went to market.

The GM variety that is planted in 89% of U.S. soy acres gets its foreign gene from bacteria (with parts of virus and petunia DNA as well). We can't know in advance if the protein produced by bacteria, never before part of the human food supply, will provoke a reaction.

As a precaution, scientists compare the new protein with a database of proteins known to cause allergies. The database lists the proteins' amino acid sequences that have been shown to trigger immune responses.

According to criteria recommended by the *World Health Organization* (WHO) and others, if the new GM protein contains sequences found in the allergen database, the GM crop is not to be commercialized and additional testing should be done.

Sections of the protein produced in GM soy are identical to known allergens, but the soybean was introduced before the WHO criteria were established, and the recommended additional tests were not conducted.

What If Bizarre Genes Start Transferring To Humans ...

If this protein in GM soybeans is causing allergies, then the situation may be made much worse by something called *horizontal gene transfer* (HGT). That's when genes spontaneously transfer from one species' DNA to another. While this happens often among bacteria, it is rare in plants and mammals.

But the method used to construct and insert foreign genes into GM crops eliminates many of the natural barriers that stop HGT from occurring. The only published human feeding study on GM foods ever conducted on GM foods showed that parts of the gene inserted into GM soy ended up transferring into the DNA of human gut bacteria.

Furthermore, the gene was stably integrated and it appeared to be producing its potentially allergenic protein. So, years after people stop eating GM soy, they may still be exposed to its risky protein, which is being continuously produced within their own intestines.

Genetic Engineering: An Exact Science... Or A Mutation Disaster Waiting To Happen?

Biotech advocates describe the process of genetic engineering as precise, in which genes-like Legos-cleanly snap into place. This is clearly a false premise. Creating a GM crop can produce massive changes

Genetically Engineered Foods: A Source of Rising Food Allergies?—CONTINUED

in the natural functioning of the plant's DNA. Native genes can be mutated, deleted, permanently turned on or off, or change their levels of protein expression.

Collateral damage may result in increasing the levels of an existing allergen, or even production of a completely new, unknown allergen within the crop. Both appear to be the case in GM soy. Levels of one known soy allergen, trypsin inhibitor, were as much as 27% higher in raw GM soy.

Cooking soybeans normally reduces the levels of trypsin inhibitor, but GM varieties appear to be more heat-resistant. Levels in cooked GM soy were nearly as high as those found in raw soy, and up to seven times higher than in cooked non-GM soy.[8] This suggests that GM soy allergen may be more likely to provoke reactions than natural varieties.

Another study verified that GM soybeans contain a unique, unexpected protein not found in non-GM soy controls. Scientists tested the protein and found that it reacted with the antibody IgE. IgE in humans plays a key role in a high proportion of allergic reactions, including those involving life-threatening anaphylactic shock. The fact that the unique protein created by GM soy interacts with IgE suggests it might also trigger allergies.

The same researchers measured the immune response of humans to soybeans using a skin-test often used by allergy doctors. Eight people reacted to GM soy. One of these did not react to non-GM soy. The sample size is small. But the implication that some people react only to GM soy is huge, and might account for the increase in soy allergies in the UK.

Eating More Herbicides In The Name Of "Progress"

By 2004, farmers used an estimated 86% more herbicide on GM soy fields compared to non-GM.[9] Higher levels of herbicide residue in GM soy might cause health problems. In fact, many symptoms identified in the UK soy allergy study are also related to glyphosate exposure.

The allergy study identified irritable bowel syndrome, digestion problems, chronic fatigue, headaches, lethargy, and skin complaints including acne and eczema, all related to soy consumption.

Symptoms of glyphosate exposure include nausea, headaches, lethargy, skin rashes, and burning or itchy skin. It is also possible that glyphosate's breakdown product AMPA, which accumulates in GM soybeans after each spray, might contribute to allergies.

GM Soy Resists Essential Protein-Digesting Enzymes

The longer proteins survive in the digestive tract, the more time they have to provoke an allergic reaction. Mice fed GM soy showed dramatically reduced levels of pancreatic enzymes.

When protein-digesting enzymes are less available, food proteins last longer in the gut, allowing more time for an allergic reaction to occur. A reduction in protein digestion due to GM soy consumption could promote allergic reactions to a wide range of proteins, not just to the soy. No human studies of protein digestion related to GM soy have been done.

Genetically Engineered Foods: A Source of Rising Food Allergies?—CONTINUED

Soy's Little-Known Link to Peanut Allergies

There is at least one protein in natural soybeans that has cross-reactivity with peanut allergies.10 This means that for those who are allergic to peanuts, eating soybeans could trigger a reaction.

It is certainly possible that the unpredicted side effects from GM soybeans might increase the incidence of this cross-reactivity. But it is unlikely that it has been researched. GM soy was introduced into the U.S. food supply in late 1996. We are left only to wonder whether this influenced the doubling of U.S. peanut allergies from 1997 to 2002.

Gambling With Our Health — For Their Profits

Introducing genetically engineered foods into our diet was done quietly and without the mandatory labeling that is required in most other industrialized countries. Without knowing that GM foods might increase the risk of allergies or which foods contain GM ingredients, the biotech industry is gambling with *our* health for *their* profit.

This risk is not lost on everyone. In fact, millions of shoppers are now seeking foods that are free from any GM ingredients. Ohio-based allergy specialist John Boyles, MD, says, "I used to test for soy allergies all the time, but now that soy is genetically engineered, it is so dangerous that I tell people never to eat it — unless it says organic."11

Organic Foods Are Not Allowed to Contain GM Ingredients

Buying products that are certified organic or that say non-GMO are two ways to limit your family's risk from GM foods.

Another is to avoid products containing any ingredients from the seven food crops that have been genetically engineered: soy, corn, cottonseed, canola, Hawaiian papaya and a little bit of zucchini and crook neck squash. This means avoiding soy lecithin in chocolate, corn syrup in candies, and cottonseed or canola oil in snack foods.

Fortunately, the *Campaign for Healthier Eating in America* will soon make your shopping easier. This Consumer Non-GMO Education Campaign is orchestrating the cleaning out of GM ingredients from foods and the natural products industry.

The campaign will circulate helpful non-GMO shopping guides to organic and natural food stores nationwide, and provide consumers with regular GM food safety updates explaining the latest discoveries about why "Healthy Eating Means No GMOs".

Jeffrey M. Smith is the author of the new publication Genetic Roulette: The Documented Health Risks of Genetically Engineered Foods, which presents 65 risks in easy-to-read two-page spreads. His first book, Seeds of Deception, is the top-rated and #1 selling book on GM foods in the world. He is the Executive Director of the Institute for Responsible Technology, which is spearheading the Campaign for Healthier Eating in America. Go to www.seedsofdeception.com to learn more about how to avoid GM foods.

Genetically Engineered Foods: A Source of Rising Food Allergies?—CONTINUED

NOTES AND REFERENCES

1. See for example, Charles Sheehan, "Scientists see spike in kids' food allergies," *Chicago Tribune,* 9 June 2006, http://www.monterey herald.com/mld/montereyherald/living/health/

2. See for example, Carl B. Johnson, Memo on the "draft statement of policy 12/12/91," January 8, 1992. Johnson wrote: "Are we asking the crop developer to prove that food from his crop is non-allergenic? This seems like an impossible task."

3. Louis J. Pribyl, "Biotechnology Draft Document, 2/27/92," March 6, 1992, www.biointegrity.org

4. Ibid.

5. Traavik and Heinemann, "Genetic Engineering and Omitted Health Research"

6. "Genetically modified foods, who knows how safe they are?" *CBC News and Current Affairs,* September 25, 2006.

7. J. Ordlee, et al, "Identification of a Brazil-Nut Allergen in Transgenic Soybeans," *The New England Journal of Medicine, March 14, 1996.*

8. Stephen R. Padgette et al, "The Composition of Glyphosate-Tolerant Soybean Seeds Is Equivalent to That of Conventional Soybeans," *The Journal of Nutrition* 126, no. 4, (April 1996); including data in the journal archives from the same study.

9. Charles Benbrook, "Genetically Engineered Crops and Pesticide Use in the United States: The First Nine Years"; *BioTech InfoNet,* Technical Paper Number 7, October 2004.

10. See for example, Scott H. Sicherer et al., "Prevalence of peanut and tree nut allergy in the United States determined by means of a random digit dial telephone survey: A 5-year follow-up study," *Journal of Allergy and Clinical Immunology,* March 2003, vol. 112, n 6, 1203-1207); and Ricki Helm et al., "Hypoallergenic Foods-Soybeans and Peanuts," Information Systems for Biotechnology News Report, October 1, 2002.

11. John Boyles, MD, personal communication, 2007.

Say No to GMOs!

With soy products, it is advised to choose only organic varieties as the non-organic soy products, (which are over 90% of sales) are *genetically modified* (GMO). This new food technology has raised enough concern among farmers and researchers alike that it has been banned in most parts of Europe and was recently forbidden in Ukiah, California, in Mendocino County.

The long term health effects of introducing various bacteria, virus and transgenic substances (e.g. fish into plants) is not known. Not allowing seeds of a plant to grow out with any reproductive capacity, binds farmers to purchase "terminator" seeds annually. Interestingly, the very foods people have the highest sensitivity to — wheat, soy, and corn — have been genetically modified for over ten years, to an all but unknowing public.

Ten Good Reasons to Buy Organic

1. **Organic products meet stringent standards.** Organic certification is the public's assurance that products have been grown and handled according to strict procedures without persistent chemical inputs.

2. **Organic food tastes great!** It's common sense — well-balanced soils produce strong, healthy plants that become nourishing food for people and animals.

3. **Organic production reduces health risks.** Many EPA-approved pesticides were registered long before extensive research linked these chemicals to cancer and other diseases. Organic agriculture is one way to prevent any more of these chemicals from getting into the air, earth and water that sustain us.

4. **Organic farms respect our water resources.** The elimination of polluting chemicals and nitrogen fertilizers, done in combination with soil conservation, protects and conserves water resources.

5. **Organic farmers build healthy soil.** Soil is the foundation of the food chain. A primary focus of organic farming is to protect and build healthy soils.

6. **Organic farmers work in harmony with nature.** Organic farmers respect the balance demanded of a healthy ecosystem: wildlife is encouraged by using permanent pastures, utilizing buffer zones, planting wildlife refuges and by protecting wetlands, forests and other natural areas.

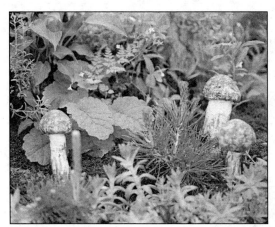

7. **Organic producers are leaders in innovative research.** Organic farmers have led the way, largely at their own expense, with innovative on-farm research aimed at reducing pesticide use and minimizing agriculture's impact on the environment.

8. **Organic producers strive to preserve diversity.** The loss of a large variety of species (biodiversity) is one of the most pressing environmental concerns. The good news is that many organic farmers and gardeners have been collecting and preserving seeds, and growing unusual varieties for decades.

9. **Organic farming helps keep rural communities healthy.** The USDA reported that in 1997, half of U.S. farm production came from only 2% of farms. Organic agriculture can be a lifeline for small farms because it offers an alternative market where sellers can command fair prices for crops.

10. **Organic abundance! Foods and non-foods alike!** Now every food category has an organic alternative. And non-food agricultural products are being grown organically — even cotton, which most experts felt could not be grown this way.

The Twelve LEAST Contaminated Fruits and Vegetables

FOOD	Twelve crops with the LEAST pesticide contamination are a good source* of the following nutrients:		SCORE**
Avocados	Vitamin A, Vitamin C, Folic Acid		7
Corn	Carotenoids, Folic Acid		14
Onions	Not a good source of vitamins or carotenoids.		18
Sweet potatoes	Potassium, Vitamin A (Carotenoids), Vitamin C		20
Cauliflower	Vitamin C		21
Brussel sprouts	Folic Acid, Vitamin A (Carotenoids), Vitamin C		36
Grapes (U.S.)	Vitamin C		40
Bananas	Potassium, Vitamin C		42
Plums	Vitamin C	(TIE)	46
Green onions	Vitamin A (Carotenoids), Vitamin C	(TIE)	46
Watermelon	Potassium, Vitamin A (Carotenoids), Vitamin C		47
Broccoli	Potassium, Vitamin A (Carotenoids), Vitamin C		49

*Includes 10% or more of the daily value of at least one of the vitamins in the contaminated food. Sources: Environmental Working Group, compiled from FDA and EPA data; Center for Science in the Public Interest, *Nutrition Action Health Letter,* January-February 1995, October 1994, May 1992, December 1991.

**200 = most toxic.

The Twelve MOST Contaminated Fruits and Vegetables

RANK	CROP		SCORE*
1	Strawberries		189
2	Bell Peppers	(TIE)	155
3	Spinach	(TIE)	155
4	Cherries (USA)		154
5	Peaches		150
6	Cantaloupe (Mexico)		142
7	Celery		129
8	Apples		124
9	Apricots		123
10	Green Beans		122
11	Grapes (Chile)		118
12	Cucumbers		117

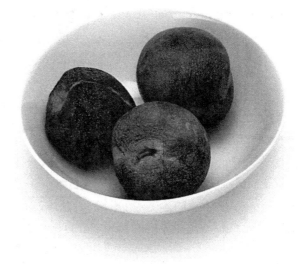

*200 = most toxic.

Appreciation of Fresh, Organic Produce

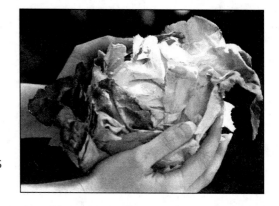

Cooking with organic produce is gaining both popularity and prestige in the culinary world. Organic produce is prized by chefs and other culinary adepts for its superb flavors when freshly picked and its superior nutritional quality.

Organic foods promote health and prevent disease when grown in an optimal environment without potentially dangerous chemical residues from pesticides and herbicides. A remarkable number of organic vegetable and fruit varieties are becoming available, each contributing its own unique flavor, color, and texture to creative culinary masterpieces.

Heirloom Vegetables

John Adams, a Washington State professor, writes:

> "When it comes to taste, the future is the past. It isn't just you. Fruits and vegetables don't taste the way they used to, and the reason they don't is the result of hybridization for safer transport and longer shelf life... the taste of open-pollinated varieties are extraordinarily different. Did you know there are 1,200 varieties of potatoes? There are hundreds of squash, beans, fruit, lettuce and nuts that no one knows about, much less has tasted."

There has always been an intimate association between the garden and the table. In the past decade, cooking with organic heirloom varieties has become very popular with restaurants, caterers, and personal chefs. Five-star restaurants such as *Chez Panisse* in Berkeley, California and the *French Laundry* in Yountville, California buy locally grown, seasonal, organic produce at peak freshness and color from community farmers with whom they have ongoing relationships, instead of from large restaurant supply grocers. Farmers' markets have sprung up all over the U.S. Gardening has become the third largest hobby in America as ever more people try their hands at backyard "kitchen gardens."

Since organic produce is becoming more popular, it should be noted that fresh foods — as perceived by researchers at Rutgers University — have an 87% higher content of magnesium, potassium, manganese, iron, and copper — since 13% of these nutrients is effectively lost when produce is shipped and stored for three or four days. We should therefore be careful to examine our packaged organic vegetables before buying.

Since there are many variables that come into play when determining whether organic produce is nutritious and flavorful, it is wise to develop your ability to assess reliable sources and select the freshest, ripest produce to buy from them.

Organic Gardening

Although organic gardening is a relatively new marketing concept, the practice of growing food organically is as old as recorded human history. Traditionally, people all over the world closely observed soil, water, weather, and natural patterns to find the optimal conditions for cultivating those crops best suited to the climate and environment of a particular place. Over generations, they selected plants with desirable attributes and saved the "open pollinating" seeds from plants whose desired characteristics came through

Appreciation of Fresh, Organic Produce—CONTINUED

each year that they were grown. Diverse cuisines — including Italian, Thai, Indian, and African — are all based on a similar principle: making good use of what Nature provides.

Gradually, chemical controls against predators, diseases, and insects became commonplace in agriculture. Chemical fertilizers and hybridized seeds became the norm. In the 1960s, the U.S. government and mega-corporations such as Monsanto — in conjunction with the United Nations — initiated a widespread agricultural program called the Green Revolution that, they proclaimed, would "end world hunger." The program introduced the American way of farming — using chemical fertilizers, pesticides, herbicides, and hybridized seeds — to countries around the world.

For ten to twenty years after farmers began to use the new methods, their productivity skyrocketed. By giving up the "old family heirlooms" and time-tested cultivation methods, they were able to grow "market-reliable" hybrids that could be sold on a larger scale. The new way was profitable and effective in solving certain insect and disease problems.

After a few decades, however, farmers began to notice insect resistance to pesticides and a sharp decline in soil fertility due to overuse of chemical fertilizers. This made heavier chemical applications and expenditures necessary. As a result, small farmers found themselves perpetually in debt. Many of them began to grow specialty crops such as sugar and wine grapes to try to make more money. Environmental and health concerns were eventually raised.

Soon the large agribusinesses were swallowing up the small farmers, making enormous profits from the sale of agricultural products by making them available to large markets on a global scale. The Green Revolution's legacy was good for small farmers in the short run, but in the long run has only served big business.

Organic Farming

In response to the economic, ecological, and health declines associated with large corporate agriculture, the organic farming movement began to emerge. Farmers found ways to work with nature, using processes that didn't exact an environmental or health price. They found that using natural methods to replenish soil fertility increased the health, vitality, and nutritional quality of their produce. Over time, a cross-pollination of ideas and methods yielded new ways of making agriculture sustainable.

Pest control methods using natural predators and products that are non-toxic to humans were developed. Methods such as French Intensive Gardening, Permaculture, and Biodynamic Gardening sprang up. Open-pollinating crops were shown to produce the same yields as the "Green Revolution" fields with a fraction of the resources, insects, and disease problems.

In California today, farmers go through a rigorous process to become certified as organic growers. Although the majority of farmers still use conventional chemical methods because they are not as labor- and knowledge-intensive, it is interesting to note that during the 1990s, marketing organic produce was the main "growth industry" in agriculture.

As a natural foods chef, you can develop relationships with the local organic farmers whose produce you purchase. They can teach you what produce is available in certain seasons, which varieties deliver the best flavors and textures, and how to ensure that your cooking is consistently local, seasonal, and organic.

Growing Organic Vegetables

Garden Produce

This can expand beyond salad gardens to include herbs, other kinds of vegetables, flowers and fruit.

French Intensive Gardening

▶ Developed by France in the 1800's when farmers moved to Paris where they had very small spaces to grow food in.

▶ Organic gardening creates an intact ecological system that does not have toxic by-products or soil-depleting practices.

▶ Farmers are the most concerned with the development and health of their soil because it is the foundation of the health and vitality within the garden.

Soil Preparation

▶ To prepare soil, take a shovel and dig a trench row along the edge of the area you want to have your garden in. Overturn the earth and pile it onto the very last part of the garden along a row.

▶ Go back to the beginning and add soil amendments such as compost, manure, potash and seaweed to the trench and dig down another 4-6 inches. Adding amendments and nutrients further develops loose, rich soil that supports closely planted crops. Mix all of this in. Then start on the next row.

▶ Take the first layer of dirt and pile it into the trench leaving a new trench in the second row. Keep going on down the line until it is all dug up. You will find the soil very soft and loose down about one foot.

▶ Making a mounding raised bed or having a frame around the garden can help to increase plant productivity and predator control.

▶ Healthy soil is formed by enzymes, bacteria, worms, insects, weather, moles and gophers. Small space and double digging loosens the soil so plant roots can penetrate deeply. The garden is ready to plant.

▶ Soil needs to be rich enough with nutrients that the plants can be grown in closer proximity and not crowd each other for their needs. Water is used more efficiently, insects are better controlled and the harvest is very fresh and delicious.

Plant Spacing

▶ Plants should be spaced in triangles. Seeds should be planted in rows with the option to thin into triangular spacing.

▶ This spacing allows the maximum amount of plants to grow together without overcrowding. Their circumference when fully grown determines the amount of space you give in between plants.

Companion Planting

▶ Plants can be planted together to complement each other such as tomatoes being planted with basil to keep away insects or onions with carrots to keep away carrot flies.

▶ Be careful to not plant certain plants together, such as fennel and beans.

Growing Organic Vegetables—CONTINUED

Cool Season Vegetables

Cool season vegetables are planted indoors in February-March or September-October and outdoors as soon as the soil is warm enough.

- ▶ Artichokes
- ▶ Asparagus
- ▶ Beets
- ▶ Broccoli
- ▶ Brussel sprouts
- ▶ Cabbage
- ▶ Cauliflower
- ▶ Celery
- ▶ Collards
- ▶ Kale
- ▶ Leeks
- ▶ Lettuce
- ▶ Mustard
- ▶ Onion

Warm Season Vegetables

Warm season vegetables are planted in March or April for midsummer to fall harvests.

- ▶ Beans
- ▶ Cantaloupe
- ▶ Carrots
- ▶ Corn
- ▶ Cucumber
- ▶ Eggplant
- ▶ Garlic
- ▶ Okra
- ▶ Parsley
- ▶ Peppers
- ▶ Potato
- ▶ Pumpkin
- ▶ Squash

Nutrient Use

- ▶ Adding organic fertilizers at certain pivotal times in the life of plants really makes a difference in vitality and productivity. You fertilize when the plant has about 3-4 sets of leaves and again every other week.

- ▶ When plants have 4-6 sets of leaves it is good to fertilize them with a high nitrogen organic fertilizer with some phosphorus and potassium in them. This can be done by mixing your own or buying it at the nursery. Make sure it is organic and not synthetic.

- ▶ You can make liquid manure — soak the manure in water overnight and then water the plants with it. Plants love it.

- ▶ Spraying seedlings with *Maxicrop*, a seaweed mix, will really bring strength and vitality to the plants. Be sure to apply the correct amount or it can burn your plants' leaves.

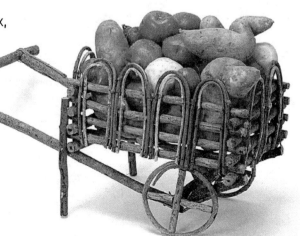

Growing Organic Vegetables—CONTINUED

Types of Nutrients

Nitrogen is the building block of proteins used by the plant to build and to create. Nitrogen comes in manures, fish emulsion, blood meal, soybean meal, green manures, alfalfa and even the rain or air. It is essential for strong growth in the newer parts of the plant. The sign of nitrogen deficiency is older leaves turning yellow and falling off at a large rate.

Phosphorus is necessary for the process of cell division, root development, resistance to disease and certain predators and the maturing fruits and seeds. Phosphorus is in bone meal, phosphate rock, and green manures. The signs of phosphorus deficiency are stunted growth and deep green leaves with yellow margins.

Potassium is a stem and structure builder and responsible for carbohydrate metabolism. The sign of potassium deficiency is weak plants with a yellow-brown mottling of the leaves, which break down. Potassium is found in wood ashes.

There are micronutrients such as *calcium, magnesium* and *sulfur* (a commonly inadequate nutrient in our Pacific West soils), *iron, zinc* and *manganese.* These can be deficient here because of the rainfall and high acidic content of the soil, especially iron which can lead to younger leaves in plants turning yellow. Changing the acidity of the soil and also adding iron can help to alleviate this problem.

Compost and Organic Soil Development

▶ One of the essential components of organic gardening is working with compost. Leaves, grass clippings, and table leftovers, can be turned into rich friable compost with a high humus content which softens the soil structure and makes nutrients more accessible to plants.

▶ To make a compost pile, dig a hole or simply start your pile in a corner of your yard. You can even put your compost pile on an area you want to eventually have a garden in. The compost actually helps to loosen the soil underneath making it easy to dig and plant in.

▶ Alternately layer dry stalks, leaves and other dry plant materials with manure and green grass clippings or fresh plant materials and food scraps. It is important to add 2-3 handfuls of manure to each layer because the manure will break down the plant material quickly. You can also add soil to the layers. Pile it up until it is 4-5 feet high. Add some water (not too much) and keep a tarp over it.

▶ Periodically turn the pile. If there is enough manure or nitrogen the pile will heat up and become hot. Turning it adds air and cools the pile down somewhat. When it is brown and sweet smelling it is ready to be put on the garden.

Heirloom Vegetables & Organic Seed Companies

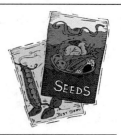

If you would like to grow vegetables, fruit and herbs to have available for cooking in your own garden, you can begin by purchasing seeds and plants from these reputable companies.

Abundant Life Seeds and Books
P.O. Box 157, Saginaw, OR 97472
541-767-9606 • www.abundantlifeseeds.com

Open pollinating vegetables as well as rare and endangered species of the Northwest.

Epicure Seeds, Ltd.
P.O. Box 23568, Rochester, NY 14692

Choice varieties of gourmet seed houses in Europe.

Gurney's
Yankton, SD 57079
513-354-1491 • www.gurneys.com

Unusual vegetables, herbs, fruit, grasses and bulbs.

Hart Seed Company
P.O. Box 6705, Hamden, CT 06517
203-776-2091 • www.yankeegardener.com

Largest selection of old-fashioned and non-hybrid vegetables. Many hard-to-find varieties available.

Johnny's Selected Seeds
955 Benton Ave., Winslow, ME 04901
207-861-3900 • www.johnnyseeds.com

Terrific seed company with integrity. Send postcard.

Redwood City Seed Company
P.O. Box 361, Redwood City, CA 94064
650-325-7333 • www.ecoseeds.com

Non-hybrid, vegetables, hot peppers and herb seed.

Renee's Garden Seeds
7389 W. Zayante Rd., Felton, CA 95018
888-880-7228 • www.reneesgarden.com

Selection of delicious varieties of vegetables and a recipe book. Originally Shepherd's Seeds.

Seeds of Change Organic Seeds
1364 Rufina Circle #5, Santa Fe, NM 8750
888-762-7333 • www.seedsofchange.com

Unique variety of vegetables, herbs, seeds, fruit trees, and books.

Seed Savers Exchange (SSE)
3076 North Winn Rd, Decorah, IA 52101
563-382-5990 • www.seedsavers.org

A non-profit organization saving old time food crops from extinction. Kent and Diane Whealy founded SSE after an elderly, terminally ill relative bestowed three kinds of garden seeds brought from Bavaria four generations earlier. They began searching for other heirloom varieties and soon discovered a vast, little-known genetic treasure.

Stark Brothers Nurseries and Orchards
P.O. Box 1800, Lousiana, MO 63353
800-325-4180 • www.starkbros.com

Specialize in fruit trees, especially dwarfs and semi-dwarfs. Carries many varieties developed by Luther Burbank.

Suttons Seeds
Woodview Road, Paignton Devon TQ4 7NG
0870-220-2899 • www.suttons-seeds.co.uk

Flowers, vegetables, bulbs and perennials for gourmet gardeners.

Swallow Tail Gardens
122 Calistoga Rd. #178, Santa Rosa, CA 95409
707-538-3585 •
www.swallowtailgardenseeds.com

Great Sonoma County resource for flower, herb, and vegetable seed.

Organic Vegetable Gardening Tips & Advice

Adapted from www.organicgardentips.com

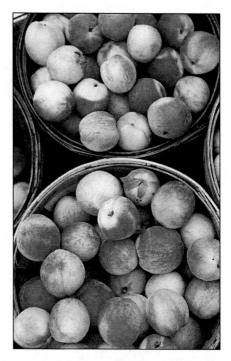

Vegetable gardening is a rewarding experience, because you end up with a delicious vegetable harvest at the end.

Garden Planning

A successful vegetable garden starts out with a plan. Planning your garden is one of the most important parts of vegetable gardening, and it's quite simple.

1. Decide what you want to grow.

2. Determine how much space you have.

3. Take a sheet of paper and draw a small scale model of your garden plot, and decide where the vegetables will go.

4. You can determine the proper distance between seeds and between rows on most seed packets. This garden measuring page shows a great way to figure out how to measure distances with your hands and feet.

Why not complement your organic yard by growing organic vegetables and herbs? Just imagine treating your taste buds to nature's own food. What do you like? Tomatoes and potatoes, cucumbers in large numbers, peas and peppers, thyme at the right time?

If you have a small yard, you can use containers for your vegetables and herbs. Containers can be found in a variety of sizes, shapes, and colors. You will undoubtedly be able find just the right containers for your needs.

Companion Planting

You probably already have a place in mind for a vegetable plot. Perhaps your herbs will have their own little section of the plot, or even a plot of their own. If you are thinking about container gardening, you probably plan to plant rosemary in one container and thyme in another. This sounds great, but there is a better way. It is called *companion planting.*

Companion planting is another way of working with nature. Some dissimilar plants have developed a symbiotic relationship-they help each other survive. Of course plants that have a similar pH should be planted together, but many symbiotic plant relationships go much farther than pH.

The most famous symbiotic relationships are *"Carrots Love Tomatoes"* and *"Roses Love Garlic".* There are many other plant relationships that you can use to enhance the beauty and health of your organic yard. Symbiotic relationships are not limited to vegetables liking vegetables, but include relationships between many different plants. You can use these relationships to enhance your vegetables and herbs, as well as other plants in your yard. Your imagination is your only limit.

Organic Vegetable Gardening Tips & Advice—CONTINUED

Types of Companion Plant Relationships

There are several kinds of plant relationships that you can use. Understanding them will help you to choose the best companion choices for your yard.

Nitrogen Fixation

Although *atmospheric nitrogen* (N2) makes up nearly 80% of our air, plants cannot use nitrogen in the N2 form. N2 is considered an inert gas because it is very stable-it is composed of two nitrogen molecules that are held together by a triple bond. Plants need ammonia, which is nitrogen combined with hydrogen (NH3), in order to manufacture amino acids, proteins, and other essentials. However, they are unable to break the N2 bond without help.

Legumes and rye are well known for their ability to 'fix' nitrogen. Actually, they both have a symbiotic relationship with various strains of Rhizobium bacteria. Rhizobium bacteria attaches itself to the roots of host plants and absorbs both nitrogen and *hydrogen* (NH2) from air in the soil and uses some of the plant's energy (carbohydrates) to change it to *ammonia* (NH3). The plant absorbs the NH3 and converts it to *ammonium nitrate* (NH4). Ammonium nitrate is a fertilizer for the plant. Both the bacteria and plant benefit from the trade-off.

If you plant oxygen-fixing legumes, such as beans or peas, near nitrogen loving members of the cabbage family, such as broccoli and kale, the cabbage family and legume family will both smile.

Repelling Pests and Attracting Help

Some plants emit chemicals from their roots or leaves, called allelochemicals, which repel pests. As an example, tomatoes repel caterpillars from diamondback moths, which like to use cabbage leaves for food.

Other plants attract insects that prey on pests that would otherwise damage nearby plants. As an example, beans attract insects that eat corn pests, such as leaf beetles.

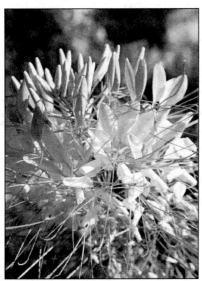

You can learn a lot more about how to fight specific pests organically at the Organic Pest Control web site: **www.organicgardenpests.com**

Space and Other Factors

Plants that need partial shade often grow best in the shade of a larger plant or bush. As an example, spider flowers (cleome) can provide the partial shade that lettuce prefers. Sometimes a row of sturdy plants can protect weaker plants from wind damage.

Root depths vary from one plant to another. You can take advantage of this difference to grow more vegetables in a given area. As an example, by planting shallow-rooted onions in close proximity to deep-rooted carrots, you can grow more of each in your vegetable garden.

Organic Vegetable Gardening Tips & Advice—CONTINUED

The Unexplained

When basil is planted in close proximity to tomatoes, both grow very well. This is a beneficial relationship that hasn't been explained.

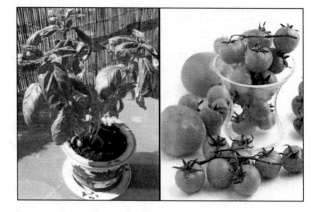

Another similar relationship is between climbing beans, corn, and squash. When the three grow together, they are all happy, but know one knows exactly why.

For more information on companion planting, visit these web sites online:

www.eap.mcgill.ca/Publications/EAP55.htm

www.ghorganics.com

Planning Your Vegetable and Herb Garden

Since many vegetables, herbs, flowers, and other plants grow very well together, be creative. Don't just think about a vegetable plot and an herb plot. Instead, think about vegetables, herbs, flowers, and more. You can even plant a vegetable garden that enhances the rest of your landscape. Nature is never this plant and that plant, but a whole variety of diverse environmental relationships.

You will certainly want a vegetable plot and herb plot, or vegetable-herb plot. You can also try planting garlic in your rose garden and nasturtium with your cabbages. Look around your yard. You might be surprised at the possible companions you can create.

Container Gardening

Container gardening may be the answer when space is limited. Containers can also be used to accentuate decks, patios, entrances, and other areas. Most vegetables and herbs can grow well in containers, especially if you pay attention to companion planting.

For more information about containers and container gardening, visit these web sites online:

www.cleanairgardening.com

www.containergardeningtips.com

Size, Light, and Other Basics

Your vegetables and herbs need a lot of sun. They should also be planted in raised beds because they need good drainage. In addition, you will need paths between the rows of vegetables so that you can work with them and harvest them.

Organic Vegetable Gardening Tips & Advice—CONTINUED

Elevating the soil between paths doesn't work very well because watering tends to flatten it again. Using wood for raised beds is better, but wood breaks down over time. Chemically treated wood lasts longer, but still breaks down over time and its chemicals leach into the soil. This is where creativity and companion planting come to the rescue.

Why does your veggie-herb patch have to be square or rectangular? Why does it have to have straight rows? Straight rows are important on a farm, but are they important in your yard? Oftentimes veggie-herb patches are hidden. They are placed out of sight near a fence or in some other area with inadequate light because they are considered unsightly. Why not think "out of the box"? You can make your vegetable and herb garden into a beautiful and colorful addition to your landscape — a showpiece.

As an example, you can make raised beds by using sculptured cement blocks — the ones that are usually used for building garden walls. There are several varieties and they can be used to create plots of almost any shape. Best of all, they won't rot.

Take some time to plan your raised bed so that it goes well with your landscape. It can even be two or more smaller raised beds. Round, oval, and kidney shapes are only a few of the possibilities. However, make sure they get plenty of sun and are not too close to trees. Tree roots often grow far beyond the drip line and can grow up into your raised bed.

Soil for Your Raised Beds

Be sure to use high quality organic soil with lots of compost in your new raised beds. The same advice goes for containers. You will also need to build up the soil each year, so be sure to begin composting with compost bins in your back yard, and maybe a compost pail for your kitchen, if don't have them already.

For instructions on composting, visit Compost Guide online at: **www.compostguide.com**

Which Vegetables and Herbs

Now you need to decide which vegetables and herbs you want to plant and where to plant them. Colors and characteristics, along with companion planting, can be used to accentuate and beautify your garden.

If you plant a crop of, say, carrots and tomatoes, don't plant them all at the same time. Instead, plant small quantities at two or three week intervals so that you can enjoy them for a longer period.

For information on specific vegetables and herbs, visit online at:

www.eap.mcgill.ca/Publications/EAP55.htm

Other Gardening Articles

We recommend **www.gardenfrog.com** for daily updated links to the best new gardening articles on the web. You can comment on each article or even submit links to gardening articles that you think everyone else should know about.

Fifty Organic Gardening Tips

Adapted from www.organicgardentips.com

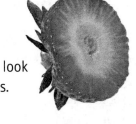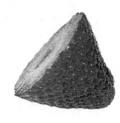

Need tips on specific types of vegetables or herbs? Just look below for vegetable gardening and herb gardening tips.

1. Mulch your flower beds and trees with 3 inches of organic material — it conserves water, adds humus and nutrients, and discourages weeds. It gives your beds a nice, finished appearance.

2. Mulch acid-loving plants with a thick layer of pine needles each fall. As the needles decompose, they will deposit their acid in the soil.

3. The most important step in pest management is to maintain healthy soil. It produces healthy plants, which are better able to withstand disease and insect damage.

4. Aphids? Spray infested stems, leaves, and buds with a very dilute soapy water, then clear water. It works even on the heaviest infestation.

5. Compost improves soil structure, texture, and areation, and increases the soil's water holding capacity. It also promotes soil fertility and stimulates healthy root development.

6. Look for natural and organic alternatives to chemical fertilizers, such as the use of compost. Our use of inorganic fertilizer is causing a toxic buildup of chemicals in our soil and drinking water.

7. When buying plants for your landscape, select well-adapted plant types for your soil, temperature range, and sun or shade exposure.

8. Landscaping your yard is the only home improvement that can return up to 200% of your original investment.

9. Plant trees! They increase in value as they grow and save energy and money by shading our houses in the summer, and letting the sun shine through for warmth in the winter.

10. Think of trees and their locations as the walls and roofs of our outdoor rooms, when you are planning their locations and sizes.

11. Grass won't grow? Find an appropriate ground cover for the exposed earth and fill the problem space, creating an interesting bed shape.

12. Plant vines on walls, fences, and overhead structures for quick shade, vertical softening, and colorful flower displays.

13. If gourmet cooking is in your plans, organically grown herbs make wonderful landscape plants. They flavor foods, provide medicinal properties, and offer up fragrances. And most thrive on neglect.

14. Shade gardens are low maintenance — they require less watering, slower growth, and fewer weeds to fight.

15. Everyone loves flowers! Annuals are useful for a splash of one-season color. But since replacing them each year is expensive, concentrate them in just a few spots.

16. There is no need to work the soil deeply when adding compost or soil amendments. Eighty-five percent of a plant's roots are found in the top 6 inches of soil.

Fifty Organic Gardening Tips—CONTINUED

17. The best organic matter for bed preparation is compost made from anything that was once alive, for example leaves, kitchen waste, and grass clippings.

18. Dig an ugly hole when planting a tree or shrub. A hole with "glazed" sides from a shovel will restrict root penetration into the surrounding soil.

19. Planting from plastic containers? Carefully remove the plant and tear the outside roots if they have grown solidly against the container.

20. Think of mulching as "maintaining the forest floor": add 1 inch to 3 inches of compost or mulch to planting beds each year.

21. Natural fertilizers, compost and organic materials encourage native earthworms. Earthworms are nature's tillers and soil conditioners, and manufacture great fertilizer.

22. Bare soil should not be visible around a new planting. Always cover with a layer of mulch, any coarse-textured, loose organic material.

23. Think "biodiversity". Using many different kinds of plants encourage many different kinds of beneficial insects to take up residence in your yard.

24. Organic pest control is a comprehensive approach instead of a chemical approach. Create a healthy biodiversity so that the insects and microbes will control themselves. Using natural products and building healthy soil is the best long-term treatment for pests.

25. Weeds? Spot-spray with common full-strength household vinegar, on a sunny day. It's an organic weed killer that's safe for you and the environment.

26. Mulch! The rain and irrigation water runs off the land, eroding and depleting your unprotected soil.

27. Residential users of synthetic fertilizers and pesticides apply more pounds per acre of these chemicals then farmers do. As these pollutants run off, they harm aquatic life and contaminate the food chain. If you keep your soil healthy, you won't require chemical fertilizers.

28. Some mulching benefits are protection of roots from the sun's heat, and protection of plant crowns from winter cold.

29. To prevent diseases and pest infestation , avoid piling mulch against tree trunks. Spread mulch out as far as the drip line.

30. For effective weed control use a layer of coarse mulch 3 inches or more in depth. Some hardy grasses may need to be rooted out for successful removal.

31. For a good start, water the ground thoroughly before and after applying a mulch cover.

32. Use plants in your landscape that are either native to your area, or were imported from areas with similar climate and soil. They require a lot less water and care, and won't die off in the winter.

33. Compost is what happens when leaves, grass clippings, vegetable and fruit scraps, woodchips, straw, and small twigs are combined, then allowed to break down into a soil-like texture. Use it instead of commercial fertilizers.

34. Formal gardens are for you if you love symmetry. They work best around a focal point like a fountain, sculpture, specimen tree, or group of plants.

Fifty Organic Gardening Tips—CONTINUED

35. Some flowers, including sweet peas, iris, foxglove, amaryllis, lantana, lupines, clematis, dature, poinsettia, and oleander, are poisonous.

36. When buying annuals or perennials, select plants that are budded but not yet in bloom, so their energy the first two or three weeks in your garden will be directed toward making larger and stronger plants with better-developed root systems.

37. To increase water conservation, look for drought-resistant plants. Usually these plants have silver leaves, deep taproots and small leaves. Succulents are also able to withstand dry weather.

38. When planting, take into consideration the plant's size at maturity. Layer by height and bloom time for emphasis and constant color.

39. Soaker hoses deliver water directly to the base of the plant, reducing moisture loss from evaporation. Early morning is the best time of day to water.

40. Compost balances both acid and alkaline soils, bringing PH levels into the optimum range for nutrient availability. It contains micronutrients such as iron and manganese that are often absent in synthetic fertilizers.

41. Avoid frequent, deep cultivation, which can damage plant roots, dry out the soil, disturb healthy soil organisms, and bring weed seeds to the surface where they will germinate.

42. Use the least-disruptive and least-polluting protections against a pest. Try the following methods as applicable: first physical removal, barriers, and traps; next, biological controls; then, appropriate botanical and mineral pesticides.

43. Red, orange, and yellow in your landscape will draw the eye and bring objects closer. To make a small garden feel larger, place warm colors in the front of the space and cool colors in the back.

44. Cover street noise — sound pollution can be minimized by the use of water features, such as a waterfall, or a pond with a fountain jet. Wind chimes also help, as can bird feeders that attract songbirds.

45. Newly planted trees need supplemental water to avoid transplant shock, so water deeply on a weekly basis throughout the growing season.

46. Give order to your garden by defining the boundaries with fences, stone walls, or hedges. Include paths for movement.

47. Less than 2% of the insects in the world are harmful. Beneficial insects such as ground beetles, ladybugs, fireflies, green lacewings, praying mantids, spiders, and wasps keep harmful insects from devouring your plants. They also pollinate your plants and decompose organic matter.

48. Plant newly purchased plants during the late evening or on a cloudy day. They have a much better chance of surviving if planted during cloudy, rainy weather than dry, sunny weather.

49. Compost introduces and feeds diverse life in the soil, including bacteria, insects, worms, and more, which support vigorous plant growth.

50. Bright light washes out the cool colors, blue, green, and purple. They are best used in shaded areas for maximum impact.

Home Deliveries of Organic Food from the Web

Most of us on the West Coast pretty much take for granted the availability of organics. Maybe you have clients, friends or family who are shut-ins, elderly, or new moms and unable to easily access healthy shopping. Or, maybe you have friends or relatives out of state — rural dwellers, and Mid-west and deep South especially — who have very limited access to organics. Whichever is the case, everyone can appreciate a chance to have a wider selection of organics to choose from.

There are "no-meat", meat, wild game, produce, body products, international offerings, cookbooks and gift ideas offered at the following web sites:

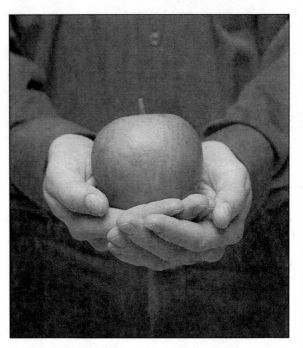

- ▶ www.bainbridgefarms.com
- ▶ www.shopnatural.com
- ▶ www.dartagnan.com
- ▶ www.nomeat.com
- ▶ www.garudainternational.com
- ▶ www.bobsredmill.com
- ▶ www.localharvest.org

This particular company offers overnight delivery of fresh produce, probably the hardest thing to find outside of California and New York:

- ▶ www.diamondorganics.com

APPENDIX ONE:
Local Organic Food Sources

In the olden times, men (and women) were known as hunters and gatherers. Nowadays, we have changed into bargain shoppers, online purchasers, fast food foragers, and reservation makers for upscale restaurants. Searching out good food sources is important; in fact, it determines how well our families will be nourished.

Fortunately, there are natural food stores and markets in many towns and cities. Organic, natural foods and supplements is the fastest growing sector in the food industry. Even commercial supermarkets are setting up organic sections in their stores.

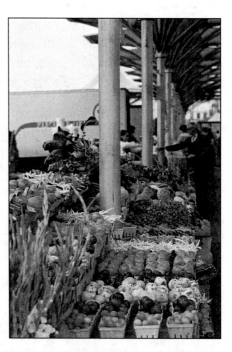

With time and practice, you can find out who in your area has the healthiest food for sale at the best price. Once that is established, share this information with your friends and associates, because the bigger the market for healthy, organic foods, the more reasonable the prices become. Meanwhile, buying food in bulk or by the case can save a great deal of money and allow for the storing and sharing of great food.

The best part of searching out local organic food sources is the opportunity to get to know the folks in your area who are growing, shipping, and selling it. Most are friendly and love to share their stories about how they got into the business. There may be family farmers in your area who at one time grew commercially and then realized that organic was the way to grow. They stand behind their produce and products, knowing that the foods they provide will create health and inner peace for those who consume it.

Connecting with local organic food sources creates a powerful, mutually beneficial, interconnected community. Food is a great way to bring people together to look at local issues and advocate for change.

As we do business with local independent stores and farmers, we support them in growing their businesses and feeding their families. In the process, we break free of the cultural obsession with fast, cheap, convenient (and addictive) food. When we know how the food was grown and handled, we can feel gratitude pervade our being as we sit down to enjoy a whole foods meal shared with friends and families.

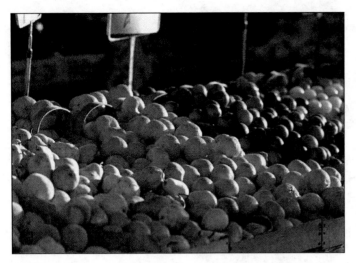

Farmers' Markets

Farmers' markets are a return to village life. Growers and their families pick the food that day and truck it into town to sell to eager shoppers. It's easy to see who has the best goods. Sampling of the foods is common. Conversation about the varieties of the fruits, vegetables and prepared foods is fun and informative. By shopping the farmers' market, we are supporting our local growers to continue to grow the best organic foods that the area will support. Buying locally saves enormously on transportation costs, fuel costs, petroleum costs and lowers pollution from burning carbon fuels. Many farmers' markets have music, art, and educational resources that create a culture of health and bring folks together around positive, joyful and healthful activities. If you have information about natural food stores and farmers' markets in your area, please forward them to Bauman College, and we will share them on our website and in updates of these *Special Edition Reports.*

One of the most enjoyable parts of traveling out of the United States to lesser-industrialized countries is that people buy their food from vendors on the streets or in open-air markets. Nearly every day, the rich and poor go to the market to purchase their food for the day from folks they know and enjoy interacting with. It's very gratifying to buy food from the people who grew it and brought it to the market. This same relationship can be cultivated at the farmers' market.

Natural food sellers are proud of their offerings. At the markets, they display the food in bushel baskets or on counters that remind me of they way they grew in the field, in plots and in bunches. Tasting food is a great part of going to a farmers' market. Each variety of apple, peaches, carrots, beets or basil has a different scent, feel, taste and experience. You can experiment with different varieties by buying small amounts. See what is ripe and then go hunting in cookbooks to see what you can do with it.

Freshness is what makes eating farmers' market food sublime. The same freshness and quality is not as likely to be found at a supermarket, where in many cases, the food is held prisoner in plastic wrap, or sprayed incessantly with water and anti-fungals.

In Northern California, the farmers' markets run six months a year or more. There is a different farmers' market nearly every day of the week. If you aren't growing your own food, then the farmers' market is the best way to get ripe, seasonal food. Some farmers' markets have fish, eggs, milk products, breads, herbs, spices, and flowers in addition to fresh produce. Get out of the big box stores and visit your local farmers' market where people and food have room to breathe and share in nature's bounty.

Sonoma County Farmers' Markets

MARKET LOCATION	DAY	TIME	MONTHS	CONTACT
CLOVERDALE FARMERS' MARKETS				
Broad Street and Cloverdale Blvd.	Sat.	9AM–11AM	June–November	707-894-3984
Franklin and South Cloverdale Blvd.	Sun.	10AM–12:30PM	June–October	
COTATI FARMERS' MARKET				Karen Silva
La Plaza Park, Downtown Cotati	Thur.	4:30PM–7:30PM	June–Sept. 15th	707-769-1830
GUALALA FARMERS' MARKET				
Gualala Community Center	Sat.	10AM–12:30PM	Memorial Day	Donna Bishop
Corner of Hwy. 1 and Center Street			- October 31st	707-884-3276
GUERNEVILLE FARMERS' MARKET				
Downtown Guerneville Park and Ride	Wed.	4PM–7PM	May 11–October 26	707-865-9380
HEALDSBURG FARMERS' MARKET				
West Plaza Parking at North and Vine	Sat.	9AM–Noon	May–December	Renee Kiff
Matheson Street on the Plaza	Tues.	4PM–6:30PM	June–October 21st	707-431-1956
MONTE RIO FARMERS' MARKET				
Parking lot across from Rio Theatre	Sat.	11am–3pm	May 28–October 29	707-865-9380
OAKMONT FARMERS' MARKET				Hilge Schwartz
Oakmont Drive and White Oak	Sat.	9AM–Noon	Year-round	707-538-7023
OCCIDENTAL FARMERS' MARKET				
Downtown in front of Howard Station	Fri.	4PM–Dusk	June–October 28th	707-793-2159
PETALUMA FARMERS' MARKETS				
Walnut Park	Sat.	2PM–5PM	May–October 29th	Erika Burns-Gooder
Petaluma Blvd. South at D Street				707-762-0344
Downtown Plaza	Sun.	10AM–1PM	June–October	
McKinley St. at Petaluma Ave				
RINCON VALLEY FARMERS' MARKETS				
Rincon Valley Community Center	Wed.	9AM–Noon	May–November	
Montecito Blvd.				
4th Street and E Street, Santa Rosa	Thur.	5PM–8:30PM	May–September	
SANTA ROSA ORIGINAL MARKET				
Veteran's Memorial Building	Sat.	8:30AM–Noon	Year-round	
Maple St. and Highway 12	Wed.	8:30AM–Noon	Year-round	
SANTA ROSA FARMERS' MARKETS				
4th St. between B St. and D St.	Wed.	5PM–8:30PM	May–August 31ST	707-524-2123

Sonoma County Farmers' Markets—CONTINUED

MARKET LOCATION	DAY	TIME	MONTHS	CONTACT
SEBASTOPOL FARMERS' MARKET Downtown Plaza at McKinley Street	Sun.	10AM–1:30PM	April-November	Paula Downing 707-522-9305
SONOMA FARMERS' MARKETS Arnold Field, Sonoma Depot Park at First Street West Sonoma Plaza on the Square	Fri. Tue.	9AM–Noon 5:30PM–Dusk	Year-round April-October	Hilge Schwartz 707-538-7023
WINDSOR FARMERS' MARKET Town Green in Old Downtown Windsor	Sun. Thur.	10AM–1:30PM 5PM–8PM	May-November	707-433-4595

Marin County and Napa County Farmers' Markets

MARKET LOCATION	DAY	TIME	MONTHS	CONTACT
CORTE MADERA CERTIFIED FARMERS' MARKET Tamalpais Drive at Hwy 101 Town Center Central Courtyard	Wed.	Noon–5PM		Manager: Lynn Bagley (415) 382-7846
FAIRFAX CERTIFIED FARMERS' MARKET Broadway and Pacheco, in Fairfax Theatre Parking Lot	Wed.	4PM–8PM	June-Sept	Manager: Marin County Farmers' Market Assoc. (800) 897-FARM
LARKSPUR CERTIFIED FARMERS' MARKET Larkspur Landing Circle, Larkspur	Sat.	10AM–2PM	May-Oct	Manager: Lynn Bagley (415) 382-7846
MARIN CIVIC CENTER CERTIFIED FARMERS' MARKET Civic Center, San Rafael	Sun. Thur.	8AM–1PM 8AM–1PM	All Year All Year	Manager: Marin County Farmers' Market Assoc. (800) 897-FARM
NAPA CHEF'S CERTIFIED FARMERS' MARKET Corner of First and Main, Napa	Fri.	4PM–8PM	May-Aug	707-252-7142
NAPA DOWNTOWN CERTIFIED FARMERS' MARKET In the COPIA parking lot, adjacent to 500 First St.	Tue.	7:30AM–12PM	May-Oct	707-252-7142
OLD TOWN NOVATO CERTIFIED FARMERS' MARKET Grant Ave., Novato	Tue.	4PM–8PM	May-Oct	Manager: Marin County Farmers' Market Assoc. (800) 897-FARM
POINT REYES CERTIFIED FARMERS' MARKET 11250 Hwy. 1, Point Reyes Station	Sat.	9AM–1PM	June-Oct	Manager: Marin Organic (415) 663-9667

Marin County and Napa County Farmers' Markets—CONTINUED

MARKET LOCATION	DAY	TIME	MONTHS	CONTACT
SAN GERONIMO VALLEY FARMERS' MARKET Valley Presbyterian Church	Sat.	9:30AM-1:30PM	May-Oct	Manager: Diane Matthew (415) 488-4746
DOWNTOWN SAN RAFAEL CERTIFIED FARMERS' MARKET Fourth Street between B and Cijos, San Rafael	Thur.	6PM-9PM	April-Sept	Manager: Brigitte Moran (415) 457-2266
SAUSALITO CERTIFIED FARMERS' MARKET Sausalito Ferry Landing, Bridgeway and Tracy	Fri.	4PM-8PM	May-Oct	Manager: Lynn Bagley (415) 382-7846
ST. HELENA-NAPA VALLEY CERTIFIED FARMERS' MARKET Crane Park on Crane Avenue	Fri.	7:30AM-11:30AM	May-Oct	707-486-2662

East Bay Farmers' Markets

MARKET LOCATION	DAY	TIME	MONTHS	CONTACT
ALAMEDA FARMERS' MARKET Taylor and Webster Streets, Alameda, CA	Tue. Thur.	9:30AM-1PM 4PM-8PM	Year-round June 9-September 8	800-949-3276
BERKELEY FARMERS' MARKET Center Street and M.L.K. Jr. Way Derby Street and M.L.K. Jr. Way Shattuck Ave. and Rose	Sat. Tue. Thur.	10AM-3PM 2PM-7PM 2PM-7PM	Year-round Year-round All-organic	510-548-3333
EAST OAKLAND FARMERS' MARKET Faith Deliverance Church 73rd Avenue and International Blvd.	Fri.	10AM-2PM	April-December	510-638-1742
EL CERRITO FARMERS' MARKET San Pablo and Fairmont	Tue./Sat.	9AM-1PM	Year-round	510-528-7992
FREMONT/CENTERVILLE MARKET Bonde Way and Fremont Blvd.	Sat.	9AM-1PM	June-November	800-897-3276
FREMONT/IRVINGTON MARKET Bay St. and Fremont Blvd., Fremont	Sun.	9AM-1PM	Year-round	800-897-3276
GRAND LAKE FARMERS' MARKET Lakepark Way between Grand and Lakeshore, Oakland, CA	Sat.	9AM-2PM	Year-round	800-897-3276
HAYWARD FARMERS' MARKET Main and B Street, Hayward, CA	Sat.	9AM-1PM	Year-round	800-897-3276

East Bay Farmers' Markets—CONTINUED

MARKET LOCATION	DAY	TIME	MONTHS	CONTACT
JACK LONDON SQ. FARMERS' MARKET Embarcadero and Broadway Jack London Square, Oakland	Sun. Wed.	10AM-2PM 10AM-2PM	Year-round May 11-October 26	800-949-3276
KAISER HOSPITAL FARMERS' MARKET 3553 Whipple Road, Union City 39400 Paseo Padre Pkwy. Fremont 3801 Howe Street, Oakland, CA	Tue. Thur. Fri.	10AM-2PM 10AM-2PM 10AM-2PM	Year-round Year-round Year-round	800-949-3276
NORTH SHATTUCK FARMERS' MARKET 1607 Shattuck Ave., Berkeley, CA	Thur.	3PM-7PM	Year-round	510-548-3333
OLD OAKLAND FARMERS' MARKET Ninth Street and Washington St.	Fri.	8AM-2PM	Year-round	510-745-7100
PINOLE FARMERS' MARKET Fernandez Ave. and Pear St.	Sat.	9AM-1PM	May 7-November 19	800-949-3276
PLEASANT HILL FARMERS' MARKET Trelany Road behind City Hall	Sat.	10AM-2PM	May-October	925-431-8361
PLEASANTON FARMERS' MARKET West Angela St. and Main St.	Sat. 1st Wed.	9AM-1PM 6PM-9PM	Year-round May to September	800-949-3276
RICHMOND FARMERS' MARKET 325 Civic Center Plaza	Fri.	11AM-5PM	Year-round	510-758-2336
ROSSMOOR FARMERS' MARKET Rossmoor Village Clubhouse 1001 Golden Rain Rd., Walnut Creek	Fri.	9AM-11AM	May-October	800-806-3276
SAN LEANDRO FARMERS' MARKET Bayfair Mall, Fairmont and East 14th	Sat.	9AM-1PM	Year-round	800-806-3276
UNION CITY FARMERS' MARKET Cesar Chavez Park, 3871 Smith St.	Sat.	9AM-1PM	Year-round	800-949-3276
WALNUT CREEK FARMERS' MARKETS Broadway and Lincoln Avenue Bonanza and Locust	Sun. Thur.	8AM-1PM 4PM-8PM	Year-round June-October	925-431-8361
WEST OAKLAND FARMERS' MARKET Seventh Street and Mandela Pkwy.	Sat.	10AM-4PM	Year-round	510-534-7657

Santa Cruz County Farmers' Markets

MARKET LOCATION	DAY	TIME	MONTHS	CONTACT
APTOS FARMERS' MARKET Cabrillo College parking lot 6500 Soquel Drive, Aptos	Sat.	7AM–Noon	Year-round	831-728-5060
CAPITOLA FARMERS' MARKET Esplanade Dr. next to Esplanade Park Capitola Beach, Capitola	Thur.	2:30PM–6:30PM	May-September	831-454-0566
FELTON FARMERS' MARKET St. John's Catholic Church parking lot Hwy. 9 and Russell Ave., Felton www.feltonfarmersmarket.org	Tue.	2:30PM–6:30PM	May-November	831-566-7159
LIVE OAK FARMERS' MARKET E. Cliff Drive and 17th St., Santa Cruz www.santacruzfarmersmarket.org	Sun.	10AM–2PM	May-October	831-454-0566
SANTA CRUZ FARMERS' MARKET Lincoln and Cedar Streets, Santa Cruz www.santacruzfarmersmarket.org	Wed.	2:30PM–6:30PM	Year-round	831-454-0566
UC SANTA CRUZ FARMERS' MARKET Bay and High St., Santa Cruz	Tue. Fri.	12PM–6PM 12PM–6PM	June-October June-October	831-459-3240
WATSONVILLE FARMERS' MARKET Peck Street, Next to Plaza Downtown Watsonville	Fri.	3PM–7PM	Year-round	831-726-7266

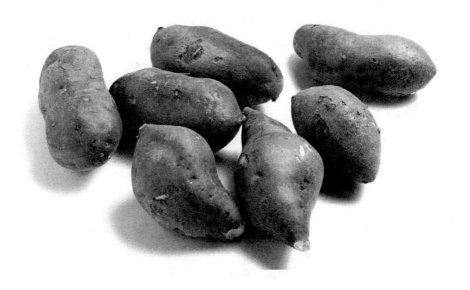

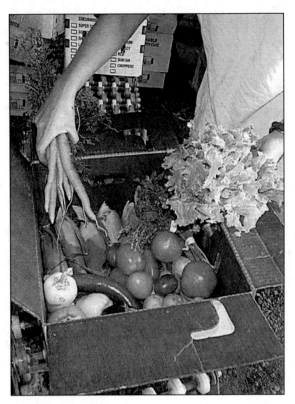

Subscription & Community Supported Agriculture (CSA)

*C*ommunity Supported Agriculture (CSA) is a new idea in farming, one that has been gaining momentum since its introduction to the United States from Europe in the mid-1980s. The CSA concept originated in the 1960s in Switzerland and Japan, where consumers interested in safe food and farmers seeking stable markets for their crops joined together in economic partnerships. Today, CSA farms in the U.S number more than 400. Most are located near urban centers in New England, the Mid-Atlantic states, and the Great Lakes region, with growing numbers in other areas, including the West Coast.

In basic terms, CSA consists of individuals who pledge support to a farmer so that his operation becomes, legally and/or spiritually, the community's farm, with the growers and consumers providing mutual support and sharing the risks and benefits of food production. Typically, members or "shareholders" of the farm or garden pledge in advance to cover the anticipated costs of the farm operation and the farmers' salary. In return, they receive shares in the farm's bounty throughout the growing season, as well as the satisfaction of reconnecting to the land and participating directly in food production.

Members also share in the risks of farming, including poor harvests due to unfavorable weather or pests. By direct sales to community members, who have provided the farmer with working capital in advance, growers receive better prices for their crops, gain some financial security, and are relieved of much of the burden of marketing.

The great part of belonging to a CSA is that a great variety locally grown foods is delivered to your doorstep each week. Alternatively, you can go directly to the farm to pick up your order and converse with other members about areas of mutual concern and delight.

Please contact each CSA directly for complete and current seasonal pickups, information and pricing.

Sonoma County Subscription and Community Supported Agriculture (CSA)

FARM LOCATION	SEASON	COST	PICKUP/DELIVERY	SPECIALTIES
CANVAS RANCH 755 Tomales Road Petaluma, CA 94952 707-766-7171 www.canvasranch.com	24-week season 4-week season	Summer: $432 Summer: $80	June-November	Vegetables, free-range Araucana eggs, honey, herbs, cashmere, fruit, flowers, honey and artisan cheese or breads.
LAGUNA FARM 1764 Cooper Road Sebastopol, CA 95472 CONTACT: Marty Falkenstein 707-823-0823 www.lagunafarm.com	Year-round	Full Share: $16/week $50 dep.	Pick up shares after 1PM Tue. at the farm or delivery Thur. afternoon to Cotati and Petaluma, Tue. to Camp Meeker, Wikkiup, E. Santa Rosa.	Members can participate in our work exchange program. Trial box available. Additional charge for home deliveries as well as fruit and bread options. Tours of the farm are available by appt.
ORCHARD FARMS 10951 Barnett Valley Rd. Sebastopol, CA 95472 CONTACT: Kenneth Orchard 707-823-6528 www.orchard-farms.com	Year round	Full Share: $18/week delivery $13/week pickup	Pickup Tue. at farm or delivered to your home in Sebastopol and Santa Rosa.	Fifty different organic vegetables strawberries, raspberries, assorted lettuces, broccoli, kohlrabi, frisee, Melons and pumpkins in the fall. Farmers' markets in Santa Rosa, Healdsburg, Oakland, and Marin.
SOL FOOD FARM 4388 Harrison Grade Rd. Occidental, CA 95472 CONTACT: Brandon Pugh 707-874-2300 www.solfoodfarm.org solfoodfarm@gmail.com	25-week season May-Nov.	Full Share: $750/year	Pickup Tue. or Fri. at farm, 3:00PM-7:00PM	Neighborly unique young farm, encourage you to pick your own flowers. Specialties include dry-farmed tomatoes, strawberries, beans and Asian greens.
SONOMA HERITAGE FARM 1095 Helman Lane Cotati, CA 94931 CONTACT: Jason Saling 707-544-2675 www.sonomaheritage.com	24-week season May-Nov.	Full Share: $18/week Delivery: $2/week	Pickup before 8:30AM Sunday at the farm or Windsor farmers' market 10AM-1PM.	Heirloom, bio-dynamic organic fruits and vegetables. Flower designer on site.
TERRA FIRMA FARM 25833 Hwy. 128 Winters, CA CONTACT: Valerie Engelman 530-756-2800 www.terrafirmafarm.com	Year round	Sm. box, $78/week Med. box, $104/week	Pickup at the farm. Delivery Tue. in San Francisco, Sacramento and Davis; Thur. in Vacaville; Fri. in Winters.	Quarterly and yearly discounts. Serving San Francisco, East Bay, Vacaville, Winters, Sacramento, Davis and Marin with certified organic vegetables and fruit.
TIERRA VEGETABLES Airport Blvd. between Fulton and Hwy. 101, Santa Rosa 1-888-TIERRA www.tierravegetables.com	30-week season	Full Share: $18/week	Pickup Tue. and Thur. at the farm stand or various drop-off sites in Santa Rosa, Healdsburg, and Windsor.	Very diverse box of vegetables and fruit. Honey, eggs, Shetland sheep wool and yarn available. Farmers' markets in Healdsburg and Ferry Plaza in San Francisco.

Please contact each CSA directly for complete and current seasonal pickups, information and pricing.

Marin County and Napa County Subscription and Community Supported Agriculture (CSA)

FARM LOCATION	SEASON	COST	DELIVERY	SPECIALTIES
GRANDPA JACK'S FARM 707-287-7366 CONTACT: Brad/Cynthia Morgan grandpajacksfarm@sbcglobal.net	Year-round	$50 bi-weekly $100/mo. 4 boxes $275 3 mo. $550 6 mo. $900 1 year	Weekly home delivery	Specializing in heirloom and unusual vegetable varieties, fresh free-range eggs, organic vegetables, melons and occasional surprises like homemade pies and Thanksgiving turkeys.
ORGANIC ABUNDANCE Napa, CA 707-251-5500 www.organicabundance.com service@organicabundance.com	Year-round	$26.95 med. box $39.95 large box	Weekly or bi-weekly delivery	Specializing in a constantly changing mix of in-season fruits and vegetables.
PARADISE VALLEY PRODUCE P.O. Box 382 Bolinas, CA 94924 CONTACT: Dennis or Sandra Dierks 415-868-0205 sdierks@marin.marin.k12.ca.us	Year-round		Weekly	Fruit, berries, vegetables, greens, potatoes, beets and herbs.

Please contact each CSA directly for complete and current seasonal pickups, information and pricing.

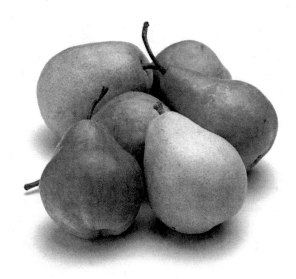

East Bay Subscription and Community Supported Agriculture (CSA)

FARM LOCATION	SEASON	COST	PICKUP/DELIVERY	SPECIALTIES
CATALÁN'S LAUGHING ONION FARM P.O. Box 1252 Hollister, CA 95024 CONTACT: Maria Catalán 831-210-1170	Year-round	Weekly boxes available.	Delivery Tue. in Berkeley/S.F.; Wed. in Salinas, Carmel, Pacific Grove, and Monterey; Sunday in San Jose.	Serving Salinas, Carmel, Monterey, Pacific Grove, San Jose, San Francisco, and Berkeley with organic vegetables, fruit, flowers, and culinary herbs.
COVELO ORGANIC VEGETABLES 23090 Hopper Lane Covelo, CA 95428 CONTACT: Tom Palley 707-983-6562 www.greenmac.com/coveg coveloov@sonic.net	25 weeks June to mid-Nov.	$15/wk. Reg. box Pickup $20/wk. Reg. box Delivered	Delivery Tues. in central Mendocino, Wed. in coastal Mendocino, and Sat. in Berkeley.	Serving Willits, Ukiah, Ft. Bragg, Mendocino, Covelo, Berkeley, Oakland and the East Bay with organic vegetables, melons, flowers, and culinary herbs.
EATWELL FARM 5835 Sievers Road Dixon, CA 95620 866-627-2465 www.eatwell.com organic@eatwell.com	Year-round	Share: $84/4 wk. $252/13 wk.	Delivery Wed. to various sites. Pickup by customer.	Serving San Francisco, Oakland, Berkeley, San Rafael, Marin, and Davis with organic vegetables, fruit, and culinary herbs. Sell at farmers' markets at S.F. Ferry Plaza, Oakland Grand Lake, and Marin.
FARM FRESH TO YOU 23808 State Hwy. 16 Capay, CA 95607 CONTACT: Kathleen Barsotti 800-796-6009 www.farmfreshtoyou.com	Year-round	$29 Reg. Mix Box $21.50 Sm. Mix Box $29 Mostly Fruit Box	Delivery throughout Bay area.	Serving San Francisco, Berkeley, Oakland, San Bruno, Alameda, Milbrae, Moraga, Orinda, Peninsula down to Palo Alto, Hwy. 4 to Discovery Bay with organic vegetables, fruit, flowers, and culinary herbs.
FROG HOLLOW FARM HAPPY CHILD CSA P.O. Box 2110 Brentwood, CA 94513 CONTACT: Alison Russum 888-779-4511 www.froghollow.com csa@froghollow.com	Year-round	$35/10 lb. Box Fruit $20/5 lb. Box Fruit	Delivery on Tue. and Sat. at S.F. Ferry Plaza and Berkeley farmers' markets, Wed. Downtown Santa Cruz farmers' market.	Serving San Francisco, Berkeley, East Bay, Marin, Palo Alto with certified organic fruits.

Please contact each CSA directly for complete and current seasonal pickups, information and pricing.

East Bay Subscription and Community Supported Agriculture (CSA)—CONTINUED

FARM LOCATION	SEASON	COST	PICKUP/DELIVERY	SPECIALTIES
FULL BELLY FARM P.O. Box 220 Guinda, CA 95637 FAX: 530-796-2199 www.fullbellyfarm.com csa@fullbellyfarm.com	Year-round	$17/week	Delivery Tue. Wed. and Fri. in East Bay; Wed. and Sat. in Davis and Sacramento, Thur. in San Rafael, Sat. on the peninsula.	Serving Yolo County, Contra Costa, East Bay, Peninsula with organic vegetables, fruit, flowers, almonds, walnuts, and wool. Home delivery Tue. and Wed. in East Bay for $5/wk.
LIVE POWER COMMUNITY FARM 25451 E. Lane Covelo, CA 95428 CONTACT: Gloria Decater 707-983-8196 www.livepower.org	30-week season	Weekly baskets available	Delivery to drop off sites in Mendocino, Marin, S.F. and East Bay. Distribution from those sites by members.	Serving bio-dynamic vegetables, fruit, eggs, grains, and chickens. Flower shares are also available.
RIVERDOG FARM P.O. Box 42 Guinda, CA 95637 CONTACT: Trini Campbell 530-796-3802 www.riverdogfarm.com csa@riverdogfarm.com	Year-round	$16/1week $208/13wk.	Delivery Tue. and Wed. 3-7PM for all sites.	Serving South Sonoma Co., Napa Co., St. Helena Co., Napa Co., Marin Co., El Sobrante to Oakland with organic vegetables and fruit.
TERRA FIRMA FARM 25833 Hwy. 128 Winters, CA CONTACT: Valerie Engelman 530-756-2800 www.terrafirmafarm.com	Year round	Sm. box, $78/week Med. box, $104/week	Pickup at the farm. Delivery Tue. in San Francisco, Sacramento and Davis; Thur. in Vacaville; Fri. in Winters.	Quarterly and yearly discounts. Serving San Francisco, East Bay, Vacaville, Winters, Sacramento, Davis and Marin with certified organic vegetables and fruit.
WINTER CREEK GARDENS 2823 Rumsey Canyon Rd. Rumsey, CA 95679 CONTACT: Chelsea Becker 530-724-3484 www.wintercreek-gardens.com	Year-round	$13/1wk. $52/4wk. Sm. box $20/1wk. $80/4wk. Lg. box	Delivery Tue. and Fri. to Davis, Sacramento and Carmichael; Wed. to Marin, S.F. and Oakland. Pickup Thur. and Sun. Civic Center San Rafael and Oakland Grand Lake farmers' markets.	Serving San Rafael, Mill Valley, S.F. Piedmont, Oakland, Davis, Sacramento, and Carmichael with certified organic herbs, flowers, fruit, melons and vegetables.

Please contact each CSA directly for complete and current seasonal pickups, information and pricing.

Santa Cruz County Subscription and Community Supported Agriculture (CSA)

LOCATION	SEASON	COST	PICKUP/DELIVERY	SPECIALTIES
CAMP JOY GARDEN 131 Camp Joy Road Boulder Creek, CA 95006 CONTACT: Jim Nelson 831-338-3651 www.campjoygarden.org	22-week season	Full Shares: $500 Flower Share: $176	Pickup on front porch of farm house.	Non-profit educational organization offering kids classes, summer camp, and a farm apprenticeship program. Serving San Lorenzo valley fruits veg etables, greens melons, and flowers.
FAN TAN FARMS 337 Golf Club Drive Santa Cruz, CA 95060 CONTACT: Jane Freedman 408-429-2246	29 week season	Full Shares: $450	Delivery in Santa Cruz.	Santa Cruz women-owned farm selling produce to many upscale organic Bay Area restaurants, including Chez Panisse in Berkeley.
HIGH GROUND ORGANICS 521 Harkins Slough Rd. Watsonville, CA 95076 831-786-0286 www.highground-organics.com csa@highground-organics.com	36 week season March -Nov.	Shares: $20/week Veg only $26/week Veg and Flowers	Delivery Wed. to Peninsula, Santa Cruz and Silicon Valley.	Members must sign up for a minimum of 9 weeks, four-week trial membership for new members. Organic vegetables, fruit and flowers.
HOMELESS GARDEN PROJECT P.O. Box 617 Santa Cruz, CA 95061 831-426-3609 www.homelessgarden-project.org	26-29 wk. season	Full Shares: $450 Half Shares: $200	Delivery in Santa Cruz.	Offers job training for homeless men and women, and scholarship shares for low-income people. Organic vegetables, fruit, and culinary herbs, Includes long-lasting flowers grown on site.
LIVE EARTH FARMS P.O. Box 3490 Freedom, CA 95019 CONTACT: Thomas Broz 831-763-2448 www.liveearthfarm.com farmers@cruzio.com	30 week season March–November	Family Share: $25/week Sm. box Half Shares: $19/week Extra Fruit: $7/week	Delivery in Santa Cruz and Monterey counties, as well as San Jose.	Members must sign up for a minimum of 9 weeks, four-week trial membership for new members. Organic vegetables, fruit and flowers.
UC SANTA CRUZ FARM AND GARDEN 1156 High Street Santa Cruz, CA 95054 CONTACT: Nancy Vail 831-459-4661	22 week season June-Oct.	Full Shares: $600 Half Shares: $350	Pickup at the farm on UC Santa Cruz campus.	Diverse organic vegetables fruit and culinary herbs. Low-income shares through a grant program. Farm tours, potlucks, harvest festivals, flower and herb cutting garden open to members.

Please contact each CSA directly for complete and current seasonal pickups, information and pricing.

Santa Cruz County Subscription and Community Supported Agriculture (CSA)—CONTINUED

LOCATION	SEASON	COST	PICKUP/DELIVERY	SPECIALTIES
MARIQUITA FARM P.O. Box 2065 Watsonville, CA 95077 CONTACT: Andy Griffin 831-761-8380 www.mariquita.com farm@mariquita.com	36 week season March – November	$80/4 wk. + flowers $104/4 wk. $180/9 wk. + flowers $234/9 wk. $691/36 wk. + flowers $898/36 wk.	Delivery on Wed. in Peninsula, and Silicon Valley; Thur. in Santa Cruz, Monterrey, Gilroy, Salinas, and Morgan Hill.	Members must sign up for a minimum of 9 weeks, four-week trial membership for new members. Organic vegetables, greens, culinary herbs, flowers, and strawberries.
TWO SMALL FARMS P.O. Box 2065 Watsonville, CA 95077 831-786-0625 www.twosmallfarms.com csa@twosmallfarms.com	36 week season March – November	$80/4 wk. + flowers $104/4 wk. $180/9 wk. + flowers $234/9 wk. $691/36 wk. + flowers $898/36 wk.	Delivery on Wed. in Peninsula, and Silicon Valley; Thur. in Santa Cruz, Monterrey, Gilroy, Salinas, and Morgan Hill.	Members must sign up for a minimum of 9 weeks, four-week trial membership for new members. Organic vegetables, greens, culinary herbs, flowers, and strawberries.

Please contact each CSA directly for complete and current seasonal pickups, information and pricing.

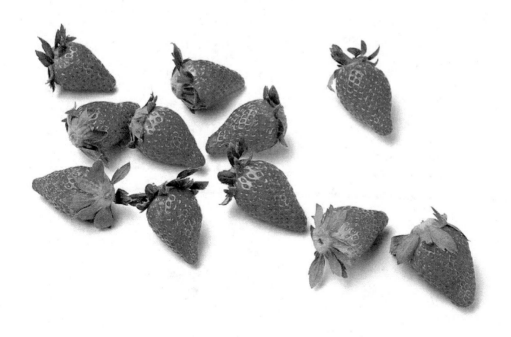

Organic Markets & Groceries

When you go to a natural market, get to know the produce people, the fish and game staff and ask them about where the food comes from, when it came to the store and what they have found to be the best picks of the day. The store staff will welcome your interest and it will allow them to become better informed about the food quality, safety and sourcing.

Sonoma County Organic Markets

ORGANIC MARKET	LOCATION
Andy's Produce	1691 Gravenstein Hwy. No., Sebastopol
Bill's Farm Basket	10315 Bodega Hwy., Sebastopol
Bohemian Market	Main St. Occidental
Cazadero General Store	6125 Cazadero Hwy., Cazadero
Community Market	1899 Mendocino Ave., Santa Rosa
Fiesta Market	550 Gravenstein Hwy. No., Sebastopol
Food For Humans	16385 1st St., Guerneville
Oliver's Market	546 E. Cotati Ave., Cotati 560 Monecito Center, Santa Rosa
Pacific Market	1465 Town and Country Drive, Santa Rosa
Pinnacle Market	Main Street, Graton
Trader Joe's	3225 Cleveland Ave., Santa Rosa 2100 Santa Rosa Ave., Santa Rosa 169 No. McDowell Blvd. Petaluma
Whole Foods Market	6910 McKinley, Sebastopol 1181 Yulupa Ave., Santa Rosa 1621 E. Washington St. Petaluma

Marin County and Napa County Organic Markets

ORGANIC MARKET	LOCATION
Andronico's Market	100 Center Blvd., San Anselmo
Bryan's Foods	341 Corte Madera Town Center, Corte Madera
Elephant Pharmacy	909 Grand Avenue, San Rafael
Golden Carrot	1621 W. Imola Ave., Napa
Good Earth Natural Foods	1966 Sir Francis Drake Blvd. Fairfax
Oasis Natural Foods	2021 Novato Blvd., Novato
Sausalito Market	46 Caledonia Street, Sausalito
Trader Joe's	337 Third Street, San Rafael 7514 Redwood Blvd., Novato 3654 Bel Aire Plaza, Napa
Whole Foods Market	414 Miller Avenue, Mill Valley 340 Third Street, San Rafael
Woodland's Market	735 College Avenue, Kentfield

East Bay Organic Markets

ORGANIC MARKET	LOCATION
Andronico's	1850 Solano Ave., Berkeley 1550 Shattuck Ave., Berkeley 1414 University Ave., Berkeley 2655 Telegraph Ave., Berkeley
Berkeley Bowl	2020 Oregon St., Berkeley
Berkeley Natural	1336 Gilman St., Berkeley 10367 San Pablo Ave., El Cerrito
Elephant Pharmacy	1607 Shattuck Ave., Berkeley
Whole Foods	3000 Telegraph Ave., Berkeley

Santa Cruz County Organic Markets

ORGANIC MARKET	LOCATION
Aptos Natural Foods	7506 Soquel Rd, Aptos
Five Mile House	2904 Freedom Blvd., Watsonville
Food Bin Herb Room	1130 Mission St., Santa Cruz
New Leaf Market	1134 Pacific Ave., Santa Cruz 1210 41st Ave., Capitola 2331 Mission St., Westside 6240 Hwy. 9, Felton 13159 Hwy. 9, Boulder Creek
Staff of Life	1305 Water St., Santa Cruz
Trader Joe's	1305 Water St., Santa Cruz 3555-D Clares St. Capitola, CA 709 Front St., Santa Cruz, CA

APPENDIX TWO:
Research Resources

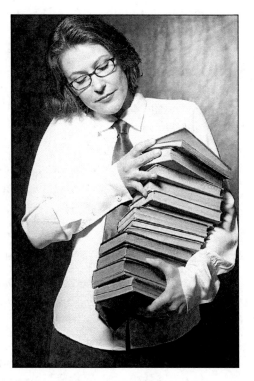

When I was a college student, doing research required an entire day or more at the college library, digging into the stacks to find reliable published information. Once I found the book or journal, I would spend hours at the photocopy machine, dropping in nickels and dimes to copy the chapters and articles I needed. Typing papers before computers came on the scene, I had to use correcto tape to clean up my mistakes. Needless to say, this was all very laborious.

Today, websites abound from universities, publications, companies, and bloggers, and information from around the globe is at our fingertips. We can readily gather information from a variety of sources and critically evaluate it for validity and reliability.

The nutrition professional is only as credible as the sources of information he provides to his clients. Bias is a major problem with web-generated information. Nutrition professionals can help consumers sort out fact from fiction so they can make informed decisions concerning food, herbs, and dietary supplements.

In this section, we provide the sources of information that we have screened and use in our work. Even with these sites, the user has to maintain a critical eye towards unproven claims or generalizations that are not supported by sound science and documented research.

As you find new and helpful sources of research, please let us know so we can keep our list updated.

Internet Resources

The Internet puts thousands of health-related websites at our fingertips. Some of them are very useful, while others are of dubious value. It is important to be discriminating when searching the web for nutrition information, so I have compiled this small sampling of reputable sites.

Please inform us of your favorite websites and we will consider adding them to this list.

Web Databases

www.christopherhobbsmedia.com

This site includes an herbal database developed by herbalist Christopher Hobbs. After a free introductory period, a "small subscription fee" is charged to help support the site.

www.healthy.net/clinic/therapy/herbal/herbic/herbs

This site is an herbal Materia Medica, where you can look up information on almost any herb.

www.ncbi.nlm.nih.gov/entrez/query.fcgi

This is the site of *PubMed*, the National Library of Medicine's searchable system. Through *PubMed*, you can search *Medline*, a database of over 11 million articles published in more than 4600 biomedical journals and magazines. (Another site, **www.medscape.com**, also provides free Medline access.)

www.ods.od.nih.gov

This site represents the *Office of Dietary Supplements* (ODS) at the National Institutes of Health, which produces the *International Bibliographic Information on Dietary Supplements* (IBIDS) database to help consumers, health care providers, educators, and researchers find credible scientific information on a variety of dietary supplements, including vitamins, minerals, and botanicals. IBIDS provides access to bibliographic citations and abstracts from published, international, scientific literature on every sort of dietary supplement.

Websites

www.biomed.lib.umn.edu

This website is the *Bio-Medical Library* for the University of Minnesota and provides references for news articles — the ones that say, "In a recent study..." without providing further information. Here you will find the full citations for journal articles that appear in the news.

www.californiahealthfreedom.org

In September 2002, history was made in California. With the unanimous support of the legislature, Governor Davis signed into law SB-577, sponsored by the *California Health Freedom Coalition* (CHFC) and authored by Senator John Burton. As of January 1, 2003, California law now recognizes the professional legitimacy of alternative and complementary health care practitioners and allows them to legally provide and advertise their services in California. CHFC now focuses on providing resources and support to practitioners and consumers of alternative health care services in California.

www.cancerdecisions.com

Both websites are produced by Ralph Moss, Ph.D., who has spent more than 20 years investigating and writing about cancer issues. He is the author of *Cancer Therapy*, *Questioning Chemotherapy*, and *The Cancer Industry*, as well as an award-winning PBS documentary, *The Cancer War.*

Internet Resources—CONTINUED

www.ccof.org

This website for the *California Certified Organic Farmers Foundation* (CCOFF), located in Santa Cruz, includes lists of all of CCOF's organic farmers, processors, handlers, packers, and retailers, as well as CCOF certified organic crops, livestock, processed products, and organic business services. Also, apprenticeship opportunities and the organization's online magazine.

www.citizens.org

Citizens for Health the nation's leading grassroots organization committed to advancing consumer access to safe food, clean water, and informed health choices. The issues it has worked on include rewriting USDA organic guidelines, passage of medical freedom legislation in nine states, licensure of alternative practitioners, and making the labeling of GMO foods mandatory.

www.citizenshealth.org

The website of *California Citizens for Health Freedom,* a non-profit natural health freedom advocacy organization maintaining an active presence in the State Capitol. This group focuses on California legislative issues, sponsors bills, testifies before committees, and monitors the thousands of bills presented each year.

www.crayhonresearch.com

This is the website of Robert Crayhon's brain research organization. It primarily advertises his seminars, books, and products, but also features useful articles and interviews with health professionals.

www.cspinet.org

The *Center for Science in the Public Interest* (CSPI) is a consumer advocacy organization whose twin missions are to conduct innovative research and advocacy programs in health and nutrition and to provide consumers with current, useful information about their health and well-being, primarily through its *Nutrition Action Healthletter.*

www.doctormurray.com

This is the internet home of Michael T. Murray, N.D., a leading authority on natural medicine and the author of several Bauman College textbooks. Murray is on the faculty of Bastyr University in Seattle, Washington and lectures throughout the country.

www.environmentalhealthnews.org

Every day, seven days a week, you'll find more than a dozen current news stories from around the nation and the world on this interactive website. Citizens can add their own news and reports.

www.greenpeople.org

A clearinghouse of eco-friendly resources, with links to home and garden products, baby products, beauty products, vegetarian restaurants, and non-profit organizations.

www.healthfreedom.net

The *American Association for Health Freedom* (formerly the *American Preventive Medical Association*) is a national advocacy organization focused specifically on federal legislation and regulations that affect our ability to use complementary and alternative therapies.

Internet Resources—CONTINUED

www.health.nih.gov

This huge website is maintained by the *National Institutes of Health* (NIH). The site contains multiple databases (including *Medline*) in which you can search for information on clinical trials, pharmaceutical drugs, health topics, demographic groups, AIDS research, and information on minority health, women's health, bioethics, etc.

www.healthyschoollunches.org

This website offers resources for schools, parents, and nutrition activists who want to see alternatives to cheeseburgers, french fries, and pizza in school cafeterias.

www.herbs.org

The home of the *Herb Research Foundation,* which calls itself:

"The world's first and foremost source of accurate, science-based information on the health benefits and safety of herbs."

Access to information on herbs requires buying a membership.

www.ivu.org/news/veg-news

This is the website of the *International Vegetarian Union,* which contains archived news stories about plant-based nutrition, health, medicine, school lunch programs, food-related environmental issues, veganism, cruelty-free products, and factory farming.

www.johnleemd.com

The website of Dr. John Lee, author of *What Your Doctor May Not Tell You About Menopause,* contains everything you need to know about natural hormones and hormone balancing for both women and men.

www.mercola.com

Alternative health promoter Dr. Joseph Mercola's website features weekly articles, product offers, his seminar schedule, and a subscription to his weekly email newsletter.

www.nccam.nih.gov

The *National Center for Complementary and Alternative Medicine* (NCCAM), a project of NIH, is the first government-supported organization (established in 1998) dedicated to researching *Complementary and Alternative Medicine* (CAM). The site includes many resources, including public health advisories on drug/herb/nutrient interactions.

www.ourstolenfuture.org

This site provides news and updates on Theo Colborn's book, *Our Stolen Future.* It focuses on studies of hormone-disrupting chemicals and their effects on plants and animals. Using hyperlinks, the site provides explanatory materials that will give you in-depth information on the role of hormones and other biological signaling systems, which can be disrupted by a growing list of industrial chemicals.

www.pcrm.org

The *Physicians Committee for Responsible Medicine* (PCRM), founded in 1985, is a nonprofit organization that promotes preventive medicine, conducts clinical research, and encourages higher standards for ethics and effectiveness in research. PCRM president Neal D. Barnard, M.D. is the author of *Turn Off the Fat Genes; Foods That Fight Pain; Eat Right, Live Longer; Food for Life;* and other books on preventive medicine.

Internet Resources—CONTINUED

www.preventcancer.com

This is the website of the *Cancer Prevention Coalition,* whose director is Samuel Epstein, M.D., author of *The Politics of Cancer, Revisited.* The site features information on avoidable carcinogen exposures and also tackles the deeply political issue of how the "war on cancer" is funded and how it operates.

www.protectingourhealth.org

A collection of peer-reviewed overviews that evaluate the medical literature linking environmental contamination to asthma, brain cancer, breast cancer, childhood leukemia, endometriosis, infertility, learning behaviors, prostate cancer, and testicular cancer. This project has been guided by physician Ted Schettler, whose books have provided convincing evidence that children's mental development can be derailed by exposure to even low levels of chemicals in the environment.

www.rachel.org

This website electronically publishes *Rachel's Environment and Health Weekly,* named for pioneering environmentalist Rachel Carson, author of *Silent Spring.* This newsletter has provided impeccably researched and documented investigative reporting of health and environmental issues since 1986 — and every issue is available online.

www.vitamincfoundation.org

This site contains everything you could possibly want to know about Vitamin C (ascorbic acid).

Online Medical Journals

► **www.ajcn.org**
American Journal of Clinical Nutrition

► **www.annals.org**
Annals of Internal Medicine

► **www.jama.ama-assn.org**
Journal of the American Medical Association

► **http://jn.nutrition.org**
The Journal of Nutrition

► **www.nejm.org**
New England Journal of Medicine

► **www.nutrition.org**
American Society for Nutrition

► **www.thelancet.com**
The Lancet

► **www.thenutritionreporter.com**
The Nutrition Reporter

► **www.tldp.com**
The Townsend Letter for Doctors and Patients

A Sampling of Useful Web Sites

WEB LOCATION	SUBJECT OR FOCUS
www.arborcom.com	Nutrition database and newsletter
www.baumancollege.org	Research Tools on Wellness Community Page
www.drkoop.com	Drug checker and many conditions described.
www.drweil.com	Dr. Andrew Weil's website
www.endocrineweb.com	Excellent Endocrine Information
www.everest2000.net/ingles/test/ayurveda.html	Doshas
www.google.com	Search Engine
www.healthcentral.com	Dr. Dean Edell's website
www.healthy.net	Free Medline
www.herbs.com	Herbal Sales and Newsletter
www.hoptechno.com	Software
www.mendosa.com/gi.htm	Glycemic Index
www.mercksource.com	Educational Tools on Systems and Conditions
www.nal.usda.gov/fnic/	Food and Nutrition Information Center
www.newhope.com	Archived articles from Delicious Magazine and others
www.nlm.nih.gov/medlineplus	News and Free Medline
www.nlm.nih.gov	National Library of Medicine
www.nutrition.about.com	General Nutrition
www.prescription2000.com	CLINICAL PEARLS Research Summaries
www.purefood.com	Hydroponics
www.soyonlineservice.co.nz	Soy Debate
www.thyroid.about.com	Excellent Thyroid Information
www.tnp.com	The Natural Pharmacy
www.vitacost.com	Access to Healthnotes, Excellent Supplement Information

Conclusion

Eating for Health™ is a moderate, sensible, and science-based approach to creating and sustaining health. It is comprised of a carefully integrated set of values that are not influenced by trendy new fad diets or exotic, overpriced specialty products that are here today and gone tomorrow.

We encourage everyone to work with a nutrition professional or to use their own good sense to experiment and find out what foods, beverages, and nutrients best fit their taste, temperament, and needs. The basis of *Eating for Health*™ is adding more and more fresh, local, seasonal, and organic foods to one's diet. Additionally, we urge you to let go of food addictions to "nutrition bandits" such as refined carbohydrates, artificial sweeteners, damaged fats, caffeine, hormone-laden commercial meat and dairy products, food additives, and preservatives.

The health and conscience of a nation depends on the quality of the food that is consumed by its leaders, who make the decisions that affect the general public. Nero fiddled while Rome burned; all the while he and others in the court were suffering from what we could call dementia from exposure to lead, food and water contamination, and a gluttonous diet. The parallels today are frightening. We need leaders who eat well, live well, think well, and work to promote the wellbeing of their people.

Advocates for *Eating For Health*™ can speak clearly and strongly, basing their confidence on the information provided by this book. As we gain more media attention, people who are not aware of the link between corrupted food and corrupted health will recognize that they have allowed themselves to become intoxicated by fast, non-nutritive food and beverages.

Conclusion—CONTINUED

It's time to wake up and reclaim our own health and the health of our planet. Information is power. Learn, practice, and teach healthy eating. Your brain and body cells will thank you for taking responsibility for your life and wellbeing. Your senses will guide you in choosing local, fresh, and ripe organic food. Your experience of the food will let you know that your nutritional needs are being met. Shopping can become a friendly excursion into a world of choices. The organic revolution gains momentum each time we make the choice to buy fresh, local and organic.

Imagine a time about twenty years in the future, when global warming has been reversed, cities have organic gardens as the center of their parks and walkways, foreign wars and terrorism are things of the past, and the water is purified in every home, restaurant, and business. Our city, state, and national leaders realize that the health of the populace depends on the quality of the food, water, and air we all take in. Even big business gets into the act by providing organic foods to its employees as a way of curbing medical costs and absenteeism. Performance soars, as does morale and creativity. School children spend an hour or more every day in the garden, where they care for the fruits, vegetables, grains, beans, herbs, and spices that will be in their lunch and snack foods.

It's a vibrant vision, not an idle dream, if enough people understand that we can heal our ills through conscious cooking and eating. Join me in this movement by imagining a healthy future, starting now.

"You may say I'm a dreamer, but I'm not the only one..."

John Lennon

About Edward Bauman, M.Ed., Ph.D.

"Nutrition is a major form of health investing. It is safer than the stock market or blind dates to hedge against the inflation of illness. When you eat poor-quality food, you are dipping into the nutrient reserves in your bones, soft tissue, organs, glands, skin, and hair. You wear the results of being overdrawn nutritionally: an unhealthy appearance, fatigue, pain, and mood disorders."

Edward Bauman, M.Ed., Ph.D.

Edward Bauman, M.Ed., Ph.D. (University of New Mexico), is the Executive Director of Bauman College. He is a ground-breaking leader in the field of whole foods nutrition, holistic health, and community health promotion. After three decades of in-depth study of worldwide health and nutrition systems, Dr. Bauman created the *Eating for Health*™ nutrition system which is the foundation of the Bauman College Nutrition and Natural Chef Training Programs.

Ed Bauman is the Director of Bauman Nutrition, a natural health clinic in Sonoma County, California, where he and his staff provide nutritional consultation to individuals, families and business groups. Their work includes a wide range of functional metabolic assessments and health research for serious health problems.

For more information visit online at:
www.BaumanNutrition.com

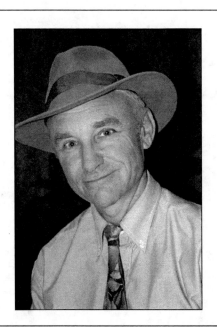

BOOKS BY
DR. EDWARD BAUMAN

▶ *Holistic Health Handbook* (1978) And/Or Press

▶ *Holistic Health Lifebook* (1980) Stephen Green Press

▶ *Holistic Health Handbook, Revised* (1984) Penguin Press

▶ *Confronting Cancer in the Community* (1999) Bauman College Press

▶ *Recipes and Remedies For Rejuvenation* (2005) Bauman College Press

▶ *Natural Chef Handbook* (2008) Bauman College Press

▶ *Nutrition Educator Handbook* (2008) Bauman College Press

▶ *Nutrition Consultant Handbook* (2008) Bauman College Press

▶ *Eating For Health*™: *Your Guide To Vitality and Optimal Health* (2008) Bauman College Press

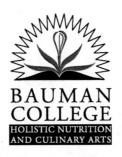